Reflexology for Women

By the same author

Thorsons Introductory Guide To Reflexology

Reflexology for Women

Nicola Hall

Thorsons
An Imprint of HarperCollins*Publishers*

Thorsons
An Imprint of HarperCollins*Publishers*
77-85 Fulham Palace Road,
Hammersmith, London W6 8JB
1160 Battery Street,
San Francisco, California 94111-1213

First published by Thorsons 1994
    3   5   7   9   10   8   6   4

A catalogue record for this book
is available from the British Library

ISBN 0 7225 2868 X

Text illustrations by Peter Cox

Phototypeset by
Harper Phototypesetters Limited, Northampton, England
Printed in Great Britain by The Bath Press, Avon

Contents

1 Introduction

Reflexology is enjoying ever increasing popularity as it is an excellent way in which to improve your health and maintain it by natural, drug-free treatment. Generally we are more health and fitness conscious than we used to be and assuming a greater role in looking after our own health and reflexology is just one of the natural means by which we can achieve the aim of good health.

Reflexology is a gentle form of natural healing that involves treatment by massage to the reflex areas, which are in the feet and hands. The reflex areas correspond to all the various parts of the body and, therefore, the method offers a means for treating the whole body. Help can be given for a wide range of disorders, including headaches, migraines, sinus congestion, stiffness in the neck and back, digestive problems, hormonal problems, heart conditions, kidney problems and many many more. Although, obviously, it is not a magical 'cure-all', most people who try reflexology treatment do find that they benefit to some degree - the problem clears up completely, the symptoms become less severe or their pain is relieved or they feel better generally in themselves. The treatment is also very relaxing and one that is pleasant to receive and these factors can only have had a positive effect on its popularity.

In addition to being able to treat all sorts of different disorders, reflexology can also be used as a means of diagnosis, to the extent that it can be used to detect which parts of the body are working well and which are not. This can often be helpful in finding the cause of a specific problem and may also help prevent other problems arising. It must be noted that reflexology cannot be used to diagnose to the extent of giving definite names to disorders, but just to the extent of establishing where imbalances exist in the body.

The following chapters will explain what the method of reflexology is about and how it can be used to help different conditions. Seeking professional treatment is always advisable, but many people do find that they are able to help themselves in the treatment of minor complaints. However, it is wise – even essential with more serious conditions – to seek professional help because in some instances treatment by this means may not be the best option and, in some instances, a person may get a little worse after treatment as the body readjusts and toxins are cleared from the system. Also, for those taking medication, there is sometimes the need for the medication to be adjusted as the reflexology treatment takes effect. These points will be mentioned again later where they apply, but it must be appreciated that the professional practitioner, having undergone thorough training, will understand the correct approach to treatment and will also work in conjunction with orthodox doctors, where necessary, and not in opposition to their advice. It must be remembered that both the reflexologist and the doctor are working to the same end – to help the patient to get better.

It seems that more women than men decide to try reflexology treatment and I am sure that most practitioners would agree that the majority of their patients are women. Most men who opt for reflexology treatment do so because their wife or girlfriend suggested it! However, the method is one that is suitable for both sexes and for all age groups, and the young through to the elderly. There are also more women reflexology practitioners than men and more women attending training courses in reflexology, either for the purpose of setting up as a professional practitioner or for gaining sufficient knowledge to be able to help themselves and their families.

Having been involved with reflexology for over 15 years, it is wonderful to see the growing interest in a method that can be so helpful to so many and without harmful side-effects. It still never ceases to give me enormous pleasure when people respond well to the treatment and are cleared of problems that, often, have been troubling them for many years. If you try reflexology treatment, then I am sure that you will not be disappointed. Included in the following pages there will be details of some of the results which myself and other practitioners have had and which will, I hope, encourage you to try reflexology for yourself, your family and your friends.

The method of reflexology is a very simple one, but it is capable of bringing about remarkably good results. I hope it does this for you.

2 What Reflexology is and Where It Came From

Reflexology in History

The method of reflexology - treating the body by massaging the feet or hands in places in a certain particular way - is, in its present-day form, a relatively new treatment. However, the origins of reflexology probably date back many years. It is thought that reflexology may have developed out of the various types of therapies first practised by the Chinese several thousands of years ago, which include methods such as acupuncture, acupressure and various other pressure therapies. Reflexology is similar to acupuncture in that the treatment is based on working on certain points along energy lines to balance the energy flow in the body, but the meridian, or energy, lines of acupuncture and acupressure differ somewhat to the energy, or zone, lines worked on in reflexology. Although there is some overlap in terms of the reflex points in the feet and hands used in reflexology and the meridian points in the feet and hands used in acupuncture and acupressure, even these are not in exactly the same places.

A tomb drawing on the tomb of Ankhmahor, dating back to 2330 BC, was found at Saqqara in Egypt and it showed two men, apparently practitioners, each holding on to another man's foot, apparently the patients, in the same manner reflexology practitioners do today, so it appears that the ancient Egyptians were also aware of a method similar to or even the same as the reflexology of today. The translation of the hieroglyphics above the scene is 'Do not let it be painful, says one of the patients. I do as you please, an attendant replies.'

Over the years it has also been established that some Red Indian tribes and some primitive tribes in Africa have been aware of reflexology and similar methods can also be traced back to India and Japan. In Europe, a book on 'zone therapy' was published by Dr Adamus and Dr A'tatis in 1582 and another book on the same subject followed shortly afterwards by a Dr Ball. It is suspected that as a result of seeing these books, an American, Dr William Fitzgerald, first became interested in zone therapy.

Zone Therapy

Dr Fitzgerald was an ear, nose and throat consultant who, in the early 1900s, became interested in various pressure therapies while studying in Europe and Great Britain. In 1917 he published the book *Zone Therapy* based on his findings. Dr Fitzgerald described how the body could be divided into longitudinal zones and that, within the zones, there was an energy flow that linked parts of the body situated in the same zone. A disturbance or energy block in a zone could affect different parts of the body situated in that zone and pressure applied to a part of the zone could help clear the energy block. In general, Fitzgerald used a variety of gadgets such as clothes pegs, metal combs and rubber bands to apply pressure within a zone, the aim being to release blocks in the energy flow in that zone. He also used the method to relieve pain and to act as an anaesthetic. Mostly the gadgets used were applied to the fingers, as the extremities of the zones, but sometimes they were applied to other parts of the zones wherever they might be on the body. The work of Fitzgerald and his contemporaries Dr Edwin Bowers and Harry Bressler did not meet with tremendous interest, but it did attract the attention of Dr Joe Riley. It is reputedly via Dr Riley that his therapist colleague, Eunice Ingham was first introduced to the method of zone therapy in the 1930s and who then went on to bring reflexology to the general public's attention.

Early Modern Reflexology

It is generally accepted that reflexology was first made known in its present-day form by an American, Mrs Eunice Ingham. She developed her work from that zone therapy described by Dr Fitzgerald. She felt that thumb and finger pressure might well be as effective if not more so than the gadgets suggested by Fitzgerald and she also thought that the feet might be a better area for pressure to be applied. The feet were, as the hands, at the extremity of the longitudinal zones and the feet were preferred to the hands because of their greater size and also because they seemed more receptive to treatment, mostly being protected by shoes and socks and so more sensitive, not being used for such a wide range of tasks as the hands. She therefore set about finding reflex areas in the feet to relate to all the parts of the body and developed 'The Ingham Method of Compression Massage'. In 1938, she published her findings in a book entitled *Stories The Feet Can Tell*. This title was shortly followed by *Stories the Feet Have Told* and these two books were the first to describe the subject of reflexology as we know it today. Eunice Ingham lectured extensively in America and, as well as treating patients, she ran training courses to teach others the method of reflexology.

In Great Britain, reflexology was first introduced by Mrs Doreen Bayly. She met Eunice Ingham while on a visit to America and was so fascinated by her work that she studied with her before returning to England to introduce the method in the 1960s. As one might expect, at this time there was not a tremendous interest in complementary therapies generally and so Doreen Bayly's work did not gain great acceptance, but she was determined to spread the word further and persevered for many years by training and teaching others. As time passed, the interest in the method grew and The Bayly School of Reflexology became established, running courses in Great Britain and Europe. In 1978, Doreen Bayly published her book *Reflexology Today* (reprinted by Healing Arts Press, Rochester, Vermont), which became a widely respected authority on the subject. Sadly, Mrs Bayly died in 1979 at a time when the great increase in interest in reflexology was just developing, but we are all indebted to her for her faith that the method would one day become much better known. The teachings of Doreen

Bayly are still continued through The Bayly School of Reflexology.

How Does It Work?

There is still, to date, no scientific explanation for why or how reflexology works. What the exact form of energy is that moves through the longitudinal zones is not known, though changes in the energy distribution around the reflex areas can be seen using Kirlian photography of the feet and the hands. The method of Kirlian photography was developed by the two Russians Semyon and Valentina Kirlian, whose work began in 1939 and was eventually given state recognition in the then USSR in the 1960s. It is a form of high voltage or electro photography and is very different to ordinary photography.

In general terms, it has been found that reflexology treatment will improve the circulation of the blood and this is beneficial because it facilitates both the better transport of necessary nutrients around the body and of waste products to the eliminatory system for removal from the body. There is also a positive effect on the nervous system as reflexology treatment helps to reduce nervous tension, which is often a root cause of a large percentage of modern illnesses.

In addition, the treatment will help to stimulate the healing forces that are already present in the body but which may not be operating. That such healing forces are present can be shown by the fact that with minor illnesses, the body can put itself right even if nothing is done to try and correct the problem - the body is continually striving to maintain itself in balance. Natural therapies, such as reflexology, can help encourage the body's own forces to go into action and often this will help speed up the recovery process.

Whether the method is working on the nervous system, the circulatory system, the endocrine system, the lymphatic system or through an energy system maybe even the same as that of acupuncture remains a subject of debate. Many theories have been put forward but none yet proven. In her book *Reflexology Today*, Doreen Bayly writes,

I believe the electrical impulse acts on the body the way the stimulus of light acts on the retina of the eye. It has been proved that the action of the full spectrum of light on the retina of the eye, in which are embedded the endings of the optic nerve, produces an electric impulse which is carried to the hypothalamus, from whence it is passed down to the pituitary gland, which passes down to lesser glands, thereby activating all the functions of the body. It is my belief that the work upon the reflexes is a parallel situation and brings about the same result.

This is but one theory.

Some say that the effect of the treatment is purely psychological in that the fact that the patient is with a caring practitioner on a one-to-one basis for about an hour and *thinks* that the treatment will help means that it *does*. Also, during this time the patient will be seated comfortably doing nothing and therefore is more likely to be relaxed and so this could explain why they feel better as a result of treatment. Certainly these ideas cannot be discounted, but other factors must be involved - these alone could not produce the recovery patients experience.

Although some scientists find it hard to accept that things do work unless there is a proven scientific reason for *why* they work, it would be foolish to cast aside a method such as reflexology on this basis alone. Whether it is working on a physical, mental or spiritual level, the excellent results that can be achieved and to which many would testify show that the method *does* work. Hopefully, in future years, proof will be found as to how it works and this should persuade those who still doubt despite the numerous positive experiences of those who have tried it and found it to be successful.

3 The Zones of the Body and the Reflexes on the Feet and Hands

The Longitudinal Zones

According to Dr William Fitzgerald, the body can be divided into longitudinal zones. He described the existence in the body of ten of these zones that divide the body into ten equal segments (see Figure 3.1). By drawing an imaginary line down the centre of the body, there are five zones on the right side of the body and five zones on the left side. These zones extend from the toes, up through the body to the head and brain and then down the arms to the fingers. The zones he described are not fine lines, like acupuncture's meridian lines, but are segments right through the body, extending from the front through to the back and, at any one level of the body, are of equal width.

He numbered the zones according to which of the toes and fingers they were in line with. Zone 1 therefore extends from the big toe up through the leg and the body to the head and brain and then down the arm to the thumb; zone 2 extends from the second toe up through the leg and the body to the head and brain and then down the arm to the second finger; zone 3 extends from the third toe up through the leg and the body to the head and brain and then down the arm to the third finger; zone 4 extends from the fourth toe up through the leg and the body to the head and brain and then down the arm to the fourth finger; zone 5 extends from the fifth, or little, toe up through the outer side of the leg and the body to the head and brain and then down the outer margin of the arm to the fifth, or little, finger. The zones have been described as running from

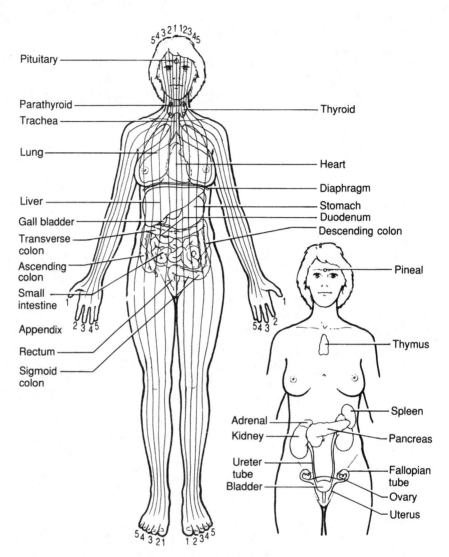

Figure 3.1 *The longitudinal zones*

the toes up the legs through the body to the head and brain and then down the arms to the fingers, but could equally well be described in reverse – as running from the fingers up the arm to the head and brain and then down through the body and the legs to the toes; the direction is not important.

The significance of the zones is that there is a flow of energy throughout each zone and this links all the areas of the body situated in the same zone. Hence, if there is a problem at one point in a certain zone of the body, this could lead to other problems involving other parts of the body situated in the same zone. This also helps to locate the position of reflex areas in the feet and the hands. As a general rule, whichever zone or zones of the body an organ is situated in, then the reflex area that corresponds to that organ will be found in the *same* zone or zones of the feet or the hands. For example, the eyes are situated in zones 2 and 3 of the body, so the reflex areas for the eyes are found in zones 2 and 3 of the feet and the hands. As the zones run longitudinally without crossing over at any point, the right foot contains reflex areas relating to parts found on the right side of the body and the left foot contains reflex areas relating to parts found on the left side of the body. Similarly, the right hand contains reflex areas for the parts found on the right side of the body and the left hand contains reflex areas for the parts found on the left side of the body. Thus, the right eye reflex area will be found in the right foot and in the right hand and the left eye reflex area will be found in the left foot and the left hand.

The Zone-related Areas

The arrangement of the longitudinal zones means that the same zones exist in both the legs and the arms and this leads to the presence in the body of what are termed *zone-related areas* (sometimes also known as *cross reflexes* or *referral areas*). The zone-related areas are shown in Figure 3.2 and are between the following areas:

- the shoulder and the hip
- the upper arm and the upper leg
- the elbow and the knee
- the forearm and the lower leg

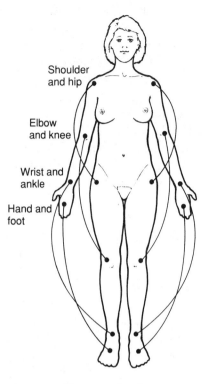

Shoulder
and hip

Elbow
and knee

Wrist and
ankle

Hand and
foot

Figure 3.2 *The zone-related areas*

- the wrist and the ankle
- the hand and the foot (the palm of the hand relating to the sole of the foot and the back of the hand relating to the top of the foot).

The zone-related areas can be most useful as additional areas for treatment for certain problems in the body. For example, in the case of tennis elbow, in addition to using reflexology through the feet or the hands, massage could be given directly to the knee as the zone-related area. If the right elbow is affected, then the right knee would be massaged; if the left elbow was affected, then the left knee would be the zone-related area. For those unskilled in massage, then direct massage to a zone-related area is safer than working directly on the affected part, which might worsen as a result. Another indication for using the zone-related areas is where there is a break or fracture. For example, if the left ankle is broken, in addition to the reflexology treatment of the relevant places on

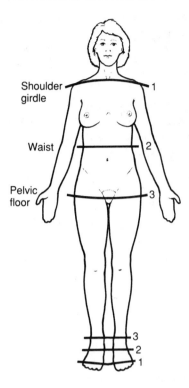

Shoulder girdle

Waist

Pelvic floor

Figure 3.3 *The transverse zones of the body*

the hands and feet, massage can be given directly to the zone-related area - in this case the left wrist - which may well help speed up the healing process and relieve pain.

The Transverse Zones

Another set of zones used in reflexology are the transverse zones and these were first described by a German practitioner, Mrs Hanne Marquardt who, like Doreen Bayly, had been a student of Eunice Ingham. These zones are particularly helpful in locating the exact positions of reflex areas in the feet.

Hanne Marquardt described the existence of three transverse zones in the body that relate to the levels of the shoulder girdle, the waist and the pelvic floor (see Figure 3.3). These zones, it was found, could be directly related to the bone structure of the foot (see Figure 3.4). The foot consists of

Figure 3.4
The transverse zones of the foot

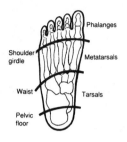

26 bones with 14 phalanges making up the toes (3 phalanges in each toe, except for the big toe, which has only 2 phalanges), 5 metatarsal bones and 7 tarsal bones. Where the phalanges meet with the next set of bones, the metatarsals, is equivalent to the level of the shoulder girdle. Working down the foot, away from the toes, where the metatarsals meet the tarsal bones is equivalent to the waist level and further down the foot again, across the tarsal bones between the ankle bones, is an imaginary line equivalent to the level of the pelvic floor.

Following on from this, the reflex areas found over the phalanges relate to areas of the body found above the level of the shoulder girdle; the reflex areas found over the metatarsal bones relate to the parts of the body found between the level of the shoulder girdle and the waist level; and the reflex areas found over the tarsal bones relate to the parts of the body found below the waist. Within the transverse zones there is no flow of energy as is found within the longitudinal zones, so the transverse zones act purely as guidelines for finding the exact position of the reflex areas in the feet. The transverse areas cannot be so neatly related to the bones that make up the hands and so are not as appropriate there.

An additional transverse zone, though not one of those described by Hanne Marquardt and not relating directly to the skeleton of the foot, is the level of the diaphragm. This area is found in the foot across the transverse arch of the foot and is found in the hand a short distance down the palm of the hand. The diaphragm level is also useful in helping to determine the exact position of reflex areas in the feet and the hands as several reflexes are positioned in the area found between the level of the diaphragm and the level of the waist.

The Reflex Areas of the Feet and Hands

Once an understanding of the arrangement of the longitudinal and transverse zones in the body and in the feet and the hands has been acquired, the position of the reflex areas can be established. It has been found that these are arranged in such a way as to form a map of the body in the feet and the hands (see Figures 3.4 and 3.5). The reflex areas described consist of reflex points that are very small - about the size of a pinhead - so accurate massage is, therefore, required, in order to work on each reflex point within a reflex area for the treatment to have any effect (the technique for this type of massage is described on page 35).

Descriptions of the positions of the various reflex areas follow below. Note that the terms 'reflex' or 'reflexes' are used to mean 'reflex areas' and 'reflex points'. Unless otherwise stated, the reflex areas will be found in similar positions in both the right and left feet and the right and left hands. Those reflexes in the right foot or hand will relate to the part found on the right side of the body and those reflexes in the left foot or hand to the part found on the left side of the body. This said, although many parts of the body are represented on *both* sides of the body, some parts are only present on *one* side, so, in such cases, the corresponding reflex areas are found in just the right foot and right hand or just the left foot and left hand as appropriate.

The Head and Brain

The head and brain areas relate to all the areas of the head, the brain, the skull protecting the brain and the scalp and the skin covering the head. The reflexes corresponding to the head and brain are found in the big toes and in the thumbs.

In the foot The reflex for the *pituitary gland* is found in the centre of the fleshy pad of the big toe. At the top of the big toe, behind the nail, is found the reflex for the *top of the head and the top of the brain* and down the side of the big toe, next to the second toe, is found the reflex for the *side of the head and the side of the brain*. The remaining parts of the big toe on the sole of the foot relate to other reflexes for the *head and brain*.

In the hand The reflex for the *pituitary gland* is found in the centre of the fleshy pad of the thumb. At the top of the thumb, behind the nail is found the reflex for the *top of the head and the top of the brain* and down the side of the thumb, next to the second finger is found the reflex for the *side of the head and the side of the brain*. The remaining parts of the thumb on the palm side relate to other reflexes for the *head and brain*.

15 ~

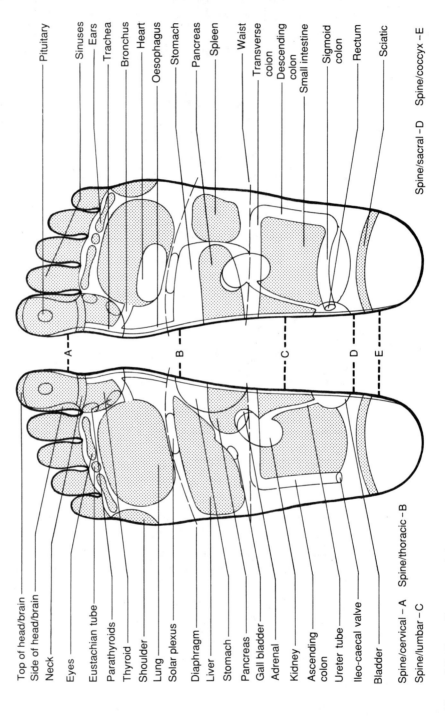

Figure 3.5 *The reflex areas of the feet and hands*

Top of head/brain
Side of head/brain
Neck
Eyes
Eustachian tube
Parathyroids
Thyroid
Shoulder
Lung
Solar plexus
Diaphragm
Liver
Stomach
Pancreas
Gall bladder
Adrenal
Kidney
Ascending colon
Ureter tube
Ileo-caecal valve
Bladder

Spine/cervical – A   Spine/thoracic – B
Spine/lumbar – C

Pituitary
Sinuses
Ears
Trachea
Bronchus
Heart
Oesophagus
Stomach
Pancreas
Spleen
Waist
Transverse colon
Descending colon
Small intestine
Sigmoid colon
Rectum
Sciatic

Spine/sacral – D   Spine/coccyx – E

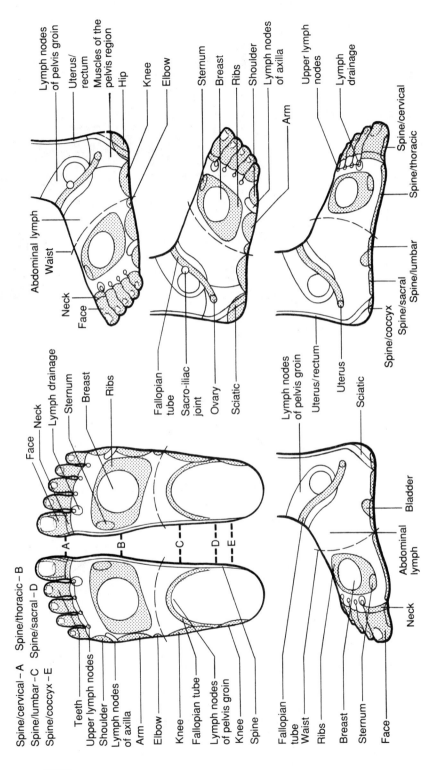

Figure 3.5 *The reflex areas of the feet and hands*

17 ❧

Spine/cervical – A   Spine/thoracic – B
Spine/lumbar – C   Spine/sacral – D
Spine/coccyx – E

Teeth
Upper lymph nodes
Shoulder
Lymph nodes
of axilla
Arm
Elbow
Knee
Fallopian tube
Lymph nodes
of pelvis groin
Knee
Spine

Face   Neck
Lymph drainage
Sternum
Breast
Ribs

Fallopian tube
Sacro-iliac joint
Ovary
Sciatic

Lymph nodes
of pelvis groin
Uterus/rectum
Uterus
Sciatic

Fallopian tube
Waist
Ribs
Breast
Sternum
Face

Abdominal lymph
Neck
Bladder

Lymph nodes
of pelvis groin
Uterus/rectum
Muscles of the
pelvis region
Hip
Knee
Elbow
Sternum
Breast
Ribs
Shoulder
Lymph nodes
of axilla
Upper lymph nodes
Lymph drainage

Abdominal lymph
Waist
Neck
Face
Arm

Spine/cervical
Spine/thoracic
Spine/lumbar
Spine/sacral
Spine/coccyx

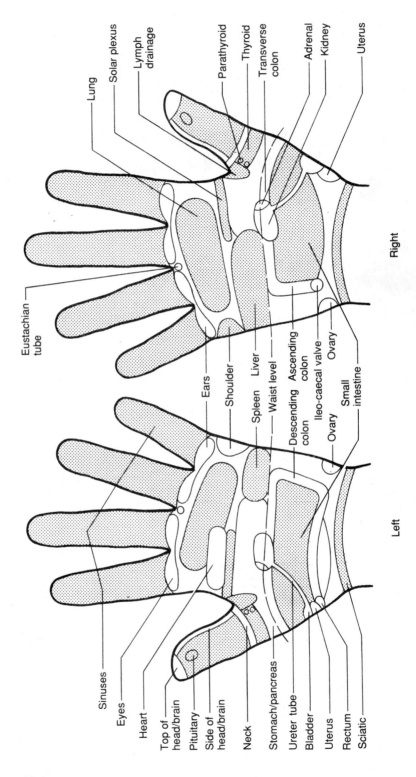

Figure 3.5 *The reflex areas of the feet and hands*

Left

Right

Lung
Solar plexus
Lymph drainage
Parathyroid
Thyroid
Transverse colon
Adrenal
Kidney
Uterus

Eustachian tube

Ears
Shoulder
Spleen
Liver
Waist level
Descending colon
Ascending colon
Ileo-caecal valve
Ovary
Ovary
Small intestine

Sinuses
Eyes
Heart
Top of head/brain
Pituitary
Side of head/brain
Neck
Stomach/pancreas
Ureter tube
Bladder
Uterus
Rectum
Sciatic

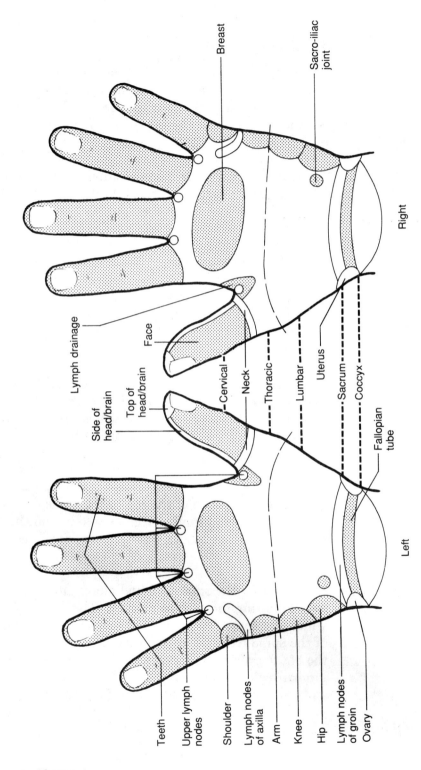

Figure 3.5 *The reflex areas of the feet and hands*

The Neck

Just as the head and brain are joined to the body by the neck area, so the big toes and the thumbs, relating to the head and brain, are joined to the foot and the hand, respectively, by the neck reflex. Rotating the big toe or thumb is equivalent to rotating the neck.

In the foot   The reflex for the *neck* is found around the base of the big toe where it joins the foot, with the back of the neck being represented in the sole of the foot and the front of the neck on the top of the foot.

In the hand   The reflex for the *neck* is found around the base of the thumb where it joins the hand, with the back of the neck being represented in the palm of the hand and the front of the neck on the back of the hand.

The Spine

The spine is made up of bony segments called vertebrae that form an important structural support for the body. Enclosed within the spinal column is the spinal cord, which is a continuation of the brain stem and so is an essential part of the nerve pathway between the brain and the other parts of the body. The spine can be divided into different regions:

- the cervical region at the top of the spine
- the thoracic and lumbar regions making up the middle
- the sacrum and coccyx (the tailbone) at the bottom of the spine.

In the foot   The reflex for the *spine* is found along the inner side of the foot, following the arch of the foot. The different regions into which the spine can be divided can be found along the length of the spine reflex, with the cervical region along the side of the big toe, then the thoracic region down to waist level, the lumbar region below waist level leading down to the sacrum and the coccyx being represented just before the heel.

In the hand   The reflex for the *spine* is found down the inner side of the hand with the cervical region along the side of the thumb, then the thoracic region down to waist level, the lumbar region below waist level leading down to the sacrum and coccyx reflex areas, which are represented just before the wrist.

The Face

The face and the areas within the face including the eyes, nose, mouth, lips and ears will all be represented by the reflex area for the face.

In the foot The reflex for the *face* is found on the front of the big toe, below the nail.

In the hand The reflex for the *face* is found on the upper surface of the thumb, below the nail.

The Sinuses

The sinuses are air-filled cavities within the bones of the skull that lighten the weight of the skull to allow the body to support it. They are lined with mucus-producing cells.

In the foot The reflexes for the *sinuses* are found up the backs and sides of the toes.

In the hand The reflexes for the *sinuses* are found up the palm side of the fingers and up the sides of the fingers.

The Teeth

The 32 teeth of the adult are important for helping break down the food eaten into smaller size particles which can be swallowed and then more readily digested. The teeth, together with the gums, are represented in the zones of the feet and hands equivalent to the zones of the body in which they are situated, with the incisors in zones 1/2, canines in zone 2, pre-molars in zone 3, molars in zone 4 and the wisdom teeth in zone 5 (little toes and little fingers).

In the foot The reflexes for the *teeth* are found on the fronts of the toes, below the nail.

In the hand   The reflexes for the *teeth* are found on the backs of the fingers, below the nail.

The Eyes

Our two eyes are the organs of sight and function together to allow light rays to be focused by the lens of the eye and directed to the back of the eye where specialized cells transmit nerve impulses to the brain to enable it to interpret what has been seen.

In the foot   The reflex for the *eyes* is found in the sole of the foot, just below where the second and third toes join the foot.

In the hand   The reflex for the *eyes* is found in the palm of the hand, just below where the second and third fingers join the hand.

The Eustachian Tubes

The Eustachian tube connects the middle ear to the throat and is important for maintaining the correct atmospheric pressure on either side of the ear-drum, which is essential for hearing.

In the foot   The reflex for the *Eustachian tube* is found in the sole of the foot, just below the web of skin between the third and fourth toes. Note that it may also sometimes be found in a similar position on the top of the foot.

In the hand   The reflex for the *Eustachian tube* is found in the palm of the hand just below the web of skin between the third and fourth fingers. Note that it may sometimes also be found in a similar position on the back of the hand.

The Ears

The ears are important for both hearing and balance. The small bones situated in the middle ear allow sound waves to be transmitted from the outer ear across to the inner ear from whence messages are passed to the hearing centres in the brain along the auditory nerve. The inner ear, as well as containing the organs of hearing, also contains areas known as semi-circular canals that help ensure that the body is aware of movements of the head and thus help it maintain balance. These areas also connect, via nerves, to the brain.

In the foot   The reflex for the *ear* is found in the sole of the foot, just below where the fourth and fifth toes join the foot.

In the hand   The reflex for the *ear* is found in the palm of the hand, just below where the fourth and fifth fingers join the hand.

The Shoulder Joints, the Arms and the Elbows

The upper limb starts with the shoulder joint where the bone of the upper arm (the humerus) joins with the shoulder blade (scapula) and collar bone (clavicle). The elbow acts as a hinge between the upper arm and forearm and the wrist joint is formed between the bones of the forearm and the hand.

In the foot   The reflex for the *shoulder joint* is found around the base of the little toe underneath the toe in the sole of the foot and on the top of the foot. Leading down from this area, along the outer side of the top of the foot, is the reflex for the *arm* and half-way down towards the heel is found the reflex for the *elbow*. The elbow reflex is actually over the slight bony projection that is often readily apparent half-way down the outer side of the foot.

In the hand   The reflex for the *shoulder joint* is found around the base of the little finger underneath the little finger in the palm of the hand and on the back of the hand. Leading down from this area along the outer side of the back of the hand is the reflex area for the *arm* and, half-way down the back of the hand towards the wrist, is found the reflex for the *elbow*.

The Thyroid Gland

The thyroid gland is situated in the front of the neck and is important for controlling the metabolic rate of the body. It also influences growth, sexual development and the level of calcium in the blood.

In the foot   The reflex for the *thyroid gland* is found around and over the ball of the big toe.

In the hand The reflex for the *thyroid gland* is found in a small area in the palm of the hand just below where the thumb joins the hand.

The Parathyroid Glands

The parathyroid glands are four small glands embedded in the back of the thyroid gland with an upper and a lower gland on each side. These glands are also important for controlling the level of calcium in the blood.

In the foot The reflexes for the *parathyroid glands* are found in the outer side of the thyroid gland area over the ball of the big toe with an upper and a lower reflex on both feet. The reflexes are, therefore, found on the edge of zone 1, next to zone 2.

In the hand The reflexes for the *parathyroid glands* are found in the outer border of the thyroid gland area in the palm of the hand just below where the thumb joins the hand with an upper and a lower reflex in both hands in the area on the edge of the thyroid gland reflex in zone 1, next to zone 2.

The Lungs

The lungs are the organs of respiration and are important for supplying the oxygen required for many processes in the body and also for eliminating carbon dioxide, a waste product of many processes in the body.

In the foot The reflex for the *lung* is found over the ball of the foot below the second, third, fourth and fifth toes.

In the hand The reflex for the *lung* is found in the palm of the hand in an area below the second, third, fourth and fifth fingers.

The Heart

The heart has the major role of pumping the blood around the body and thereby enabling areas of the body to both receive nutrients and dispose of waste products. In the body, the heart is positioned centrally in the chest region, about a third to the right side and two-thirds to the left side.

The main reflex for the heart is rather an indirect one as it does not relate straightforwardly to the same zones in which the heart is found in the body - which would be zone 1 on the right side and zones 1 and 2 on the left side. The reflex for the heart, though, is found only in the left foot and left hand.

In the foot   The reflex for the *heart* is found in the lower part of the ball of the left foot just above diaphragm level in zones 2 and 3.

In the hand   The reflex for the *heart* is found in the palm of the left hand just above diaphragm level in zones 2 and 3.

The Diaphragm

The diaphragm is a muscular band below the thoracic region of the body and is important in the process of respiration since contraction and relaxation of the diaphragm assists the lungs in the process of breathing.

In the foot   The reflex for the *diaphragm* is found across the sole of the foot in the position of the transverse arch of the foot, just below the ball of the foot.

In the hand   The reflex for the *diaphragm* is found across the palm of the hand about a quarter of the way down the palm from the fingers.

The Solar Plexus

The solar plexus is a network of nerves situated just below the diaphragm and is a useful area for helping relaxation in the body.

In the foot   The reflex for the *solar plexus* is found in zones 2 and 3, just below diaphragm level in the sole of the foot.

In the hand   The reflex for the *solar plexus* is found in zones 2 and 3, just below diaphragm level in the palm of the hand.

The Liver

The liver is the largest organ in the body and carries out a number of important functions, including storing sugars, manufacturing bile, breaking down proteins, storing vitamins, metabolizing alcohol and producing heat.

In the foot   The reflex for the *liver* is found in just the *right* foot in an area in the sole of the foot between the levels of the diaphragm and the waist. The reflex lies in all 5 zones just below the diaphragm level and then tapers off with its lower border just above waist level in zones 3, 4 and 5.

In the hand   The reflex for the *liver* is found in the palm of the right hand in an area between the levels of the diaphragm and the waist in all 5 zones just below diaphragm level and then tapering off with its lower border just above waist level in zones 3, 4 and 5.

The Gall Bladder

The gall bladder is a small pear-shaped sac attached to the lower lobe of the liver on the right side of the body and is important for storing the bile that is produced by the liver, which helps in the digestion of fats. The bile is released into the small intestine when fat is present in the food eaten.

In the foot   The reflex for the *gall bladder* is found in the sole of only the right foot in zone 3, just above waist level.

In the hand   The reflex for the *gall bladder* is found in the palm of only the right hand in zone 3, just above waist level.

The Spleen

The spleen is found on the left side of the body just above the waist. It helps to break down the old red blood cells no longer required by the body and to produce the white blood cells, called lymphocytes, that help to fight infection.

In the foot   The reflex for the *spleen* is found in the sole of only the left foot in the area between the levels of the diaphragm and the waist in zones 4 and 5.

In the hand The reflex for the *spleen* is found in the palm of only the left hand in the area between the levels of the diaphragm and the waist in zones 4 and 5.

The Stomach

The stomach is part of the digestive system. Indeed, when the food we eat reaches our stomach, it then begins to be digested.

In the foot The reflex for the *stomach* is found mainly in the sole of the left foot in the area between the levels of the diaphragm and the waist in zones 1, 2 and 3. It can also be represented in the same area in the sole of the right foot, but then just in zone 1.

In the hand The reflex for the *stomach* is found mainly in the palm of just the left hand in the area between the levels of the diaphragm and the waist in zones 1, 2 and 3. It can also be represented in the same area of the palm of the right hand, but then just in zone 1.

The Pancreas

The pancreas produces digestive enzymes that are passed to the small intestine and help in the digestion of food. It also produces hormones, including insulin, that affect the blood sugar levels. Just as in the body the pancreas is partly overlapped by the stomach, so in the feet and hands the reflex for the pancreas is partly overlapped by that for the stomach.

In the foot The reflex for the *pancreas* is found in the sole of the foot in the lower half of the area between the levels of the diaphragm and the waist. It is represented in zones 1 and 2 in the right foot and zones 1, 2 and 3 in the left foot.

In the hand The reflex for the *pancreas* is found in the palm of the hand in the lower half of the area between the levels of the diaphragm and the waist. It is represented in zones 1 and 2 in the right hand and zones 1, 2 and 3 in the left hand.

The Small Intestine

Once food has passed through the stomach, it reaches the small intestine and it is in this area that the main breakdown of food and absorption of nutrients from it takes place.

In the foot   The reflex for the *small intestine* is found in the sole of the foot in the area below the waist level but above the pad of the heel in zones 1, 2, 3 and 4.

In the hand   The reflex for the *small intestine* is found in the palm of the hand in the area between the waist level and the wrist in zones 1, 2, 3 and 4.

The Ileo-caecal Valve

The ileo-caecal valve is the valve between the ileum of the small intestine (the last part of the small intestine) and the caecum of the large intestine (the first part of the large intestine) and is found on the right side of body. The reflex for the ileo-caecal valve is therefore found where the reflexes for the small intestine and large intestine join in the right foot.

In the foot   The reflex for the *ileo-caecal valve* is found in the sole of only the right foot in zones 4 and 5, just above the pad of the heel.

In the hand   The reflex for the *ileo-caecal valve* is found in the palm of only the right hand in zones 4 and 5, just above the wrist.

The Appendix

The appendix projects off the caecum on the right side of the body and is situated very close to the ileo-caecal valve. The appendix consists of lymphatic tissue.

In the foot   The reflex for the *appendix* is found in the sole of only the right foot in zone 4, just above the pad of the heel.

In the hand   The reflex for the *appendix* is found in the palm of only the right hand in zone 4, just above the wrist.

The Large Intestine

The food not absorbed in the small intestine passes on to the large intestine to be excreted. Thus, little absorption of food substances takes place in the large intestine, but water is absorbed to prevent the body from becoming dehydrated. The large intestine is shaped rather like an incomplete rectangle around the small intestine and its reflex follows a similar pattern around the reflex for the small intestine.

In the foot The reflex for the *large intestine* is found in the soles of the feet starting with the reflex for the *ascending colon* in zones 4 and 5 on the right foot just above the pad of the heel and then passing straight upwards to waist level, where it turns through 90 degrees to become the *transverse colon* (the bend joining ascending to transverse colon is known as the hepatic flexure as it is situated just below the liver). The reflex for the *transverse colon* crosses all the zones at waist level in the right and left feet. In zones 4 and 5 on the left side, this then turns through 90 degrees to become the *descending colon* (the bend joining transverse to descending colon is known as the splenic flexure as it is situated just below the spleen). The *descending colon* reflex passes straight down in the left foot to just above the pad of the heel. It then turns across all the zones in the form of the reflex for the *sigmoid colon*. This ends in zone 1 with the reflex for the *rectum* on the inner side of the foot. There is also a reflex for the *rectum* a short distance up the back of the leg on either side of the Achilles tendon.

In the hands The reflex for the *large intestine* is found in the palms of both the right and left hands. The reflex for the *ascending colon* is found in zones 4 and 5 of the right hand, starting just above the wrist and then passing straight upwards to waist level. The reflex for the *transverse colon* then starts and crosses all the zones at waist level in the right and left hands. In zones 4 and 5 on the left side, this then becomes the *descending colon* and the reflex passes straight down in the left hand to just above the wrist. It then turns across all the zones in the form of the reflex for the *sigmoid colon*. This ends in zone 1 with the reflex for the *rectum* on the inner side of the hand. There is also a reflex for the *rectum* a short distance up the palm side of the arm from the wrist.

The Kidneys, Ureter Tubes and Bladder

The kidneys are a very important part of the body's eliminatory system and are involved in a complicated process of filtering and absorbing substances from the blood that passes through them in order to maintain the volume and composition of the body fluids. Any substances *not* required by the body are excreted by the kidneys and pass down the ureter tubes in the form of urine, which is stored in the bladder until being removed from the body.

In the foot   The reflex for the *kidney* is found in the sole of the foot at waist level in zones 2 and 3.

The reflex for the *bladder* is found on the inner side of the foot and the position is sometimes marked by a slight puffiness on the side of the foot quite close to the position of the reflex for the lumbar part of the spine. The reflex can also extend into the sole of the foot.

The reflex for the *ureter tube* crosses from the bladder reflex in zone 1 to the kidney reflex in zone 2.

In the hand   The reflex for the *kidney* is found on the palm of the hand at waist level in zones 2 and 3.

The reflex for the *bladder* is found on the inner side of the hand and slightly into the palm of the hand in zone 1, close to the reflex for the lumbar part of the spine.

The reflex for the *ureter tube* is found in the part of the palm of the hand crossing from the bladder reflex in zone 1 to the kidney reflex in zone 2.

The Sciatic Nerves

The left and right sciatic nerves are the largest nerves in the body and pass down from the lumbar and sacral regions of the spine (they arise from the lumbar and sacral nerves) across the buttock and then down the backs of the legs to the knees where they divide to supply nerves to the lower parts of the legs.

In the foot   The reflex for the *sciatic nerve* is found across the pad of the heel about one-third of the way down. In the foot, the remaining area over the pad of the heel relates to the pelvic areas. There is also a reflex for the sciatic nerve up the back of the leg for a short way on either side of the Achilles tendon.

In the hand   The reflex for the *sciatic nerve* is found across the palm of the hand just above the wrist and there is also a reflex for the sciatic nerve for a short distance up the arm from the wrist (palm side).

The Sacro-iliac Joints and Pelvic Muscles

The sacro-iliac joint is formed between the sacrum of the spine and the ilium of the pelvis. The pelvic muscles are those that sit in the pelvic region and join the areas around the lower part of the back and the top of the leg.

In the foot   The reflex for the *sacro-iliac joint* is found in a small dip just in front of the outer ankle bone in line with the fourth toe.

The reflex for the *pelvic muscles* is found in the area just below the outer ankle bone.

In the hand   The reflex for the *sacro-iliac joint* is found on the back of the hand slightly above the wrist in line with the fourth finger.

The reflex for the *pelvic muscles* is found in an area on the back of the hand above the wrist in zone 5.

The Hips and Knees

The hip joint is formed between the top of the thigh bone (femur) and the pelvis. The knee joint articulates the upper leg and lower leg. The reflexes for the hip and the knee also represent the reflexes for the upper and lower leg, respectively.

In the foot   Two half-moon shapes can be imagined on the outer side of the foot from waist level to the heel with the reflex for the *hips* being found in the first half-moon shape, just in front of the heel, and the reflex for the *knee* being found in the half-moon shape from the hip area to waist level.

In the hand   The reflexes are found on the back of the hand in the area between waist level and the wrist with the reflex for the *knee* found in the area from waist level to half-way down towards the wrist and the reflex for the *hip* being found leading down from the knee reflex to the wrist.

The Ovaries, the Fallopian Tubes and the Uterus

The ovaries, Fallopian tubes and uterus are all part of the female reproductive system.

In the foot   The reflex for the *ovary* is found on the outer side of the foot, half-way between the tip of the outer ankle bone and the back of the heel.

The reflex for the *uterus* is found on the inner side of the foot, half-way between the tip of the inner ankle bone and the back of the heel. There is also a reflex for the uterus found up the back of the leg for a short distance on either side of the Achilles tendon.

The reflex for the *Fallopian tube* is found joining the ovary and uterus areas over the top of the foot and in front of the ankle bones.

In the hand   The reflex for the *ovary* is found around the outer side of the hand, just above the wrist, on both the back and palm of the hand.

The reflex for the *uterus* is found around the inner side of the hand, just above the wrist, on both the back and palm of the hand. There is also a reflex for the uterus for a short distance up the palm side of the arm from the wrist.

The reflex for the *Fallopian tube* passes between the ovary and uterus reflexes across the back of the hand, just above the wrist.

(In males, the reflexes for the reproductive areas are represented in the same zones of the feet and the hands with the reflexes for the *testes* in the same position as the ovary reflexes. The reflex for the *prostate gland* is in the same position as the uterus reflex and the reflex for the *vas deferens* is in the same position as the Fallopian tube reflex.)

The Lymphatic System and the Breasts

The lymphatic system is rather like a secondary circulatory system in the body and is made up of lymph vessels containing a fluid similar to blood plasma called lymph. At various sites throughout the body are lymph nodes, which are collections of lymphatic tissue. The lymph nodes produce cells that purify the lymph and thus help to prevent infection occurring and spreading throughout the body. The lymphatic system is, therefore, very important as part of the defence system of the body. Eventually the purified lymph returns to the bloodstream via the subclavian veins, which are found in the neck.

In the foot   The reflexes for the *lymphatic system* are found on the top of the foot. The reflexes for the *upper lymph nodes* are found at the roots of the toes and, leading down from here on the top of the foot to above the ankles, are found the reflexes for the *thoracic and abdominal lymphatics.* Around and across the top of the ankle bones are found the reflexes for the *pelvic and groin lymphatics.* The reflex for the lymph nodes of the *axilla (armpit)* is found on the top of the foot, just below the shoulder reflex. The *lymph drainage* reflex is found below the web between the big toe and second toe. The reflex for the *breast* is found within the area for the thoracic lymphatics on the top of the foot, just above waist level, in zones 2, 3 and 4.

In the hand   The reflexes for the *lymphatic system* are found on the back of the hand. The reflexes for the *upper lymphatics* are found at the roots of the fingers and, leading down from here, on the back of the hand to the wrist, are found the reflexes for the *thoracic and abdominal lymphatics.* The reflexes for the *pelvic and groin lymphatics* are found over the wrist. The reflex for the lymph nodes of the *axilla (armpit)* is found on the back of the hand, just below the shoulder reflex. The *lymph drainage* reflex is found below the web between the thumb and the first finger. The reflex for the *breast* is found within the area for the thoracic lymphatics, just above waist level on the back of the hand in zones 2, 3 and 4.

The Skin

The skin acts as a protective barrier for the body and plays a vital role in regulating body temperature. There is not a precise reflex area relating to the skin, but, as the skin covers the whole of the body and is, therefore, present in all the zones of the body, the reflexes for particular parts of the *skin* will be found in the relevant zones of the feet and hands. Therefore, as examples, the skin of the face can be treated via the reflexes for the face and the skin of the neck can be treated through the reflexes for the neck.

In fact, for all of the areas of the body, the areas in question will relate not only to the organ, gland or joint named but also the blood supply to that area, the nerve supply to that area, the muscles around that area and the skin covering that area as these are all present in the same zones. Also, just as in the body areas overlap, so in the feet and the hands, reflexes for these areas will overlap.

From the above descriptions of the positions of the reflex areas for the main parts of the body in both the feet and hands, it can now be seen how their arrangement is a very logical one: a picture of the body appears in the feet and the hands with the various parts situated similarly there to their position in the body. Let us next look at how to massage these reflexes correctly and how it feels on the receiving end.

4 *How Treatment is Given and What is Felt*

One of the major differences between orthodox and complementary medicine is in the approach to treatment. Most complementary therapies follow an holistic approach to treatment, which means that the patient is treated as a whole rather than just their individual symptoms being treated. This is an important difference as it means treatment is far more likely to get at the root cause of a problem and treat this in addition to the symptoms and so the likelihood of the symptoms reappearing is reduced. With this in mind, therefore, it is necessary when giving reflexology treatment to treat *all* the reflex areas present in both the feet or both hands in order to treat the whole person. In this way the best results will be achieved. Also, if more than one condition is present then these can all be treated with the same treatment and often conditions that are troubling people are, in fact, interrelated. It is possible, however, to treat isolated symptoms by treating the appropriate areas in the feet or the hands, but, for the reason given earlier, this may well only bring temporary relief.

The Technique for Reflexology Massage

When giving treatment, a precise form of massage is required in order to contact each of the reflex points in the area. Mostly the thumb is used to apply the massage, holding it in a bent position (see Figure 4.1). The side *and* tip, rather than the very tip, of the thumb is applied to the reflex point using either the inner or outer side of the thumb, whichever is most comfortable. Pressure is applied to a reflex point and is

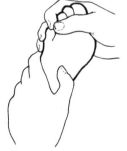

Figure 4.1
The correct angle of the thumb for treatment

maintained for a few moments, then the pressure is released. As the pressure is applied, the thumb nail is eased back against the skin of the thumb to avoid pressing the nail into the reflex point. The next reflex point is then massaged similarly. As much as possible, the thumb should be kept held in a bent position, without bending and straightening it, and should also be kept in contact with the foot or hand. The distance between reflex points within a reflex area is minute so there will be hardly any distance at all between the points where pressure is applied. Movement between points should be as smooth as possible without rubbing the skin surface and without the massage giving the impression of just prodding the different reflex points. The technique is somewhat like pressing a doorbell then releasing it just enough to allow the bell to ring but keeping the thumb on the surface of the button in case it needs to be pressed again. The pressure applied should be firm but not heavy and should be comfortable for the person giving treatment to apply without their being overly conscious of applying pressure. In some instances, the fingers are used in a similar way to apply pressure and this may be more appropriate for areas that are difficult to get at with the thumb, such as between the toes, which can be rather cramped together sometimes.

There is a considerable number of different techniques taught by different reflexology training schools, but that described above is the method that Doreen Bayly taught and it does produce very good results. Different techniques may well be effective too, but what is important is that very heavy pressure is not used on the reflex points as this is quite unnecessary and, if pain is inflicted on the patient, then the treatment will not be relaxing.

The use of gadgets to apply pressure to the reflex points is not advisable as pressure does need to be adjusted sometimes and, also, the physical touch of the practitioner's thumb or finger on a reflex point is important for healing to be effective. However, different approaches do suit different people and a certain form of reflexology used in the Far East involves pressing on the reflex points with a stick and applying a heavy pressure. In this instance, if the treatment is not really painful then the patient does not think that it has been effective!

Gadgets such as foot or hand rollers can be useful but more as exercisers for the feet and hands, helping in cases of poor circulation or tension in the feet. They may stimulate reflex areas to a degree but will not stimulate all the points evenly as, in the main, only the reflex areas in the sole of the foot or palm of the hand will be contacted and these are not the only reflex areas. The same applies to the wearing of 'reflexology sandals' and also with these there is the possibility that certain areas may be overworked as the very nature of walking means that more pressure is exerted by the foot on certain parts of the sandal. These should, therefore, be worn with care, but many wearers of these sandals do find that they are beneficial.

What Will Be Felt?

From the patient's point of view, when pressure is applied to the different reflex points in the feet or the hands, different sensations will be felt in these areas. Sometimes the patient is just aware of the pressure being applied to the foot or hand; sometimes the patient is aware of a slight discomfort - often described as a bruise-like feeling - as pressure is applied; sometimes the patient is aware of a sharpness in the foot or hand when pressure is applied and may think that the practitioner is using a fingernail on the skin.

The different degrees of comfort to discomfort felt indicate the differing imbalances in the body. In other words, the more discomfort that is felt, the more out of balance the corresponding part of the body is. Therefore, in theory, the healthy person will show no tender areas in the feet or hands but the unhealthy person will. In practice, there is considerable variation due to the fact that the sensitivity of the feet and hands varies from person to person. As a general rule, in patients with imbalances, at the very first reflexology treatment, the feet or hands are at their most sensitive, but at subsequent treatments are much less sensitive as the treatment helps to correct the imbalances. In other cases, when people first try reflexology treatment, no tender areas appear, even though the person knows that there are parts of the body not working correctly, but at the second or third treatment the feet begin to show tender areas and these then become less sensitive as a result of further treatments. There are some people who never appear to have any tender reflexes when treatment is applied, but who still benefit from the treatment and find that troublesome conditions are corrected.

The pressure applied to the reflex points has to be adjusted from one person to another to account for different levels of sensitivity. Overall, the treatment should never be unpleasant for the patient as if it is the patient will not be able to relax totally. Often people are worried that they will have very sensitive or ticklish feet, but this is very rarely the case and even those with supposedly very ticklish feet are amazed that they are able to tolerate a full reflexology treatment. The fact that the massage is given in a very definite way and not as a surprise light touch to the foot or hand accounts for the fact that it is rarely ticklish. The tender areas that are felt in the foot when pressure is applied will not normally be felt when one is walking about, even if walking barefoot.

Crystals in the Feet

In some early writings on reflexology, the method was explained as the massage of crystal deposits found in the feet, but this is not strictly the case. Sometimes when working on reflex areas in the feet, the presence of 'gritty' areas will be felt. These are often termed crystal deposits and various theories have been put forward as to what these deposits are, including calcium crystals, lactic acid crystals or uric acid crystals, but their exact composition has not ever been chemically analysed. Whatever their composition, these deposits settle at the reflex points and cause a block in the energy zone. The massage causes them to be dispersed, therefore clearing the energy blockage. They can sometimes feel like bony areas beneath the skin's surface and can, in fact, be mistaken for bone.

In addition to the tenderness felt at the reflex points in the feet or the hands, in some instances patients may actually feel a sensation in the part of the body to which the reflex point being worked on relates. This need not occur for treatment to be effective, but it can be a surprisingly clear way of proving the positions of the reflex points in the feet or hands. Also, sometimes when treatment is being given, a patient may feel a tingling sensation along the zone being worked on, which is energy flowing through the body.

Mostly, reflexology treatment is given to the feet - the hands usually only being used if the feet are not able to be worked on, such as when the foot is in plaster or when large areas of the foot are infected. The reflex areas in the feet tend to be more sensitive to reflexology massage than those in the hands, probably because they are not exposed to the elements and general wear and tear so much as the hands. The reflex areas also occupy larger areas in the feet than in the hands and so offer a larger area to be worked on. When parts of the feet cannot be worked on, then treatment is given to as much of the feet as possible and the other areas being worked via the corresponding reflexes on the hands. The hands, though, are easier to work on when treating yourself as, in most cases, people can reach the reflexes there more easily.

A Treatment Session

When visiting a reflexology practitioner for the feet to be treated, the patient is normally seated in a recliner chair or on a massage couch so that they are comfortable, with their neck, back and legs well supported. It is best that the knees are slightly bent and that the area from knee to ankle is well supported in order that the feet can be resting in a fully relaxed position.

Generally, a small amount of unperfumed talcum powder will be gently massaged onto the feet or hands at the start of treatment to enable the massage to be given more easily. The talcum will absorb any moisture or, if the feet are rather dry, it will smoothe the skin. Oils, though beneficial in general massage, are not recommended for reflexology treatment. They make the skin too slippery, making it more difficult to work precisely on the reflex points, with a tendency to slide over the points, and as it is only when there is precision in the massage that it will work, the objective of the exercise is defeated.

As the talcum is applied, the general massage to the feet

involved enables the patient to become used to the practitioner touching their feet and any tension present in the feet will begin to be reduced. Most people when they first experience a reflexology treatment will be slightly nervous about it as they will not know exactly what to expect, even if they do already have some knowledge of the subject.

A treatment session will last between 45 minutes and an hour as, during this time, all of the reflex points in both feet will need to be worked on. If the reflexes of the hands are being employed, then the length of the session will be slightly less as there is a smaller area to be worked on.

Certain reflex points will be of greater importance in certain conditions than others so extra massage will be given to these important areas. As the order of treatment is followed, a reflex area will be worked over just the once, but if it is an important area for the person in question, then this massage will be repeated two or three times before the practitioner moves on to the next area. At the very end of a treatment session, massage will again be given to these important areas and often, when going back to these areas, if any tenderness was felt previously when the area was massaged, it may have been reduced.

Order of Treatment

A specific order of treatment is normally followed to ensure that all of the reflex areas are worked on. The same order would be used for working on the feet as for working on the hands, with the whole of the right foot or right hand being treated before working on the whole of the left foot or left hand. There are many variations on the order of treatment. Some people work on the left side before the right and some work on a few points on the right and then a few on the left and vice versa. Certainly both Eunice Ingham and Doreen Bayly recommended commencing work on the right side and their advice should, I feel, be followed. To support this, by working this way the digestive tract, namely the large intestine, is worked first at the point where it starts – the ileo-caecal valve – and should thus encourage healthy elimination through this system. Also, as the heart reflex is found in the left foot, by working the right side first, the body will be in a more relaxed state before working this area, which must in any case be approached with great care. There are, however, strong reasons for following other orders, but the important thing is that all the reflex areas are worked on during a treatment session.

A Recommended Order of Treatment

Note that those areas with ⃰ after them indicate that they are found in only the *right* or only the *left* foot or hand. All of the other reflex areas are present in *both* feet and *both* hands.

RIGHT FOOT

Pituitary, neck, side of head/brain, top of head/brain, spine, face, sinuses, teeth, eye, Eustachian tube, ear, shoulder, arm/elbow, thyroid/parathyroids, lung, diaphragm/solar plexus, liver⃰, gall bladder⃰, stomach, pancreas, small intestine, large intestine (ileo-caecal valve⃰, ascending colon⃰, transverse colon), bladder, ureter tube, kidney, adrenal, sciatic loop and up back of leg, sacro-iliac joint, muscles of the pelvis, knee, hip, ovary (or testes in the male), Fallopian tube (or vas deferens in the male), uterus (or prostate in the male), lymphatics (including breast), then lymph drainage.

LEFT FOOT

Pituitary, neck, side of head/brain, top of head/brain, spine, face, sinuses, teeth, eye, Eustachian tube, ear, shoulder, arm/elbow, thyroid/parathyroids, lung, heart⃰, diaphragm/solar plexus, spleen⃰, stomach, pancreas, small intestine, large intestine (transverse colon, descending colon⃰, sigmoid colon⃰, rectum⃰), bladder, ureter tube, kidney, adrenal, sciatic loop and up back of leg, sacro-iliac joint, muscles of the pelvis, knee, hip, ovary (or testes in the male), Fallopian tube (or vas deferens in the male), uterus (or prostate in the male), lymphatics (including breast), then lymph drainage.

AFTER TREATMENT

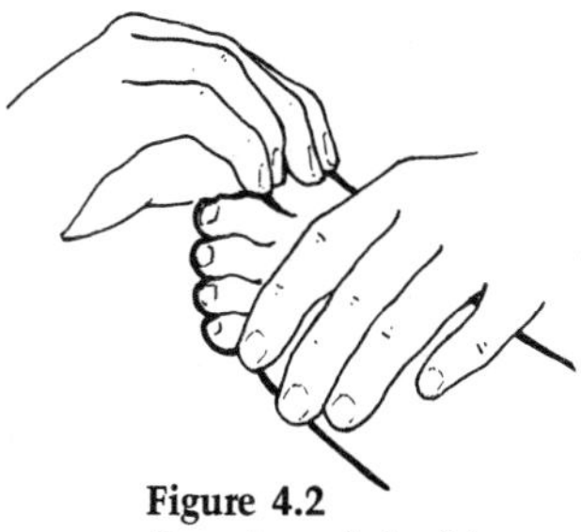

Figure 4.2
Rotation of the big toe

After giving treatment to each of the reflexes in each foot or hand, a few general exercises are carried out. These exercises are most relevant when the feet have been treated and so will be described as applied to the feet, but they can also be carried out to the hands. These exercises will include:

• *rotation of the toes* by holding the tip of each toe in turn while supporting the joint between the phalange and metatarsal (rotation of the big toe or the thumb is equivalent to rotating the neck – see Figure 4.2)

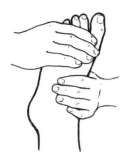

Figure 4.3
Wringing the foot

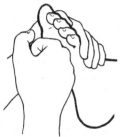

Figure 4.4
Kneading the foot

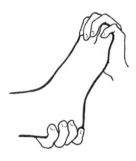

Figure 4.5
Ankle-rotation

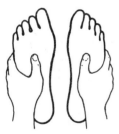

Figure 4.6
Solar plexus breathing

- *a 'wringing' action* of the foot, which is when, for the right foot, the left hand is placed around the outer side of the foot with the fingers resting on the top of the foot and the thumb underneath it and the right hand is placed further down the foot around the inner side of the foot with the fingers resting on the top of the foot and the thumb underneath it, and then the hands 'wring' the foot, spreading apart and thus spreading out the bones in the foot (for the left foot, the *right* hand is placed uppermost around the outer side of the foot and the left hand is placed lower down around the inner side of the foot - see Figure 4.3)
- *a 'kneading' action* on the foot, which is when the flat surface of a clenched fist is pressed on the foot at diaphragm level with the other hand held flat on top of the foot and the two hands, pressing towards each other from each side of the foot, are rotated around each other to knead the foot (see Figure 4.4)
- *rotation of the ankle* which is done by having one hand supporting the foot just behind the heel and the other gripping the toes and gently rotating the ankle (see Figure 4.5).

These exercises are best done after treating the reflex areas in the foot as the foot will then be in a more relaxed state and so the movements will be easier and more effective. Each of the exercises helps to reduce tension in the corresponding parts of the body. At the very end of a treatment session, a breathing exercise is carried out to finish off the treatment and to bring about further relaxation:

- *solar plexus breathing* the thumbs are placed on the solar plexus reflexes, with the right thumb on this reflex on the right foot and the left thumb on this reflex on the left foot and the fingers resting on the tops of the feet (see Figure 4.6), then, as the patient breathes in, pressure is applied to the solar plexus reflexes and the feet eased gently up towards the patient; after a deep breath and as the patient breathes out, the pressure is released and the feet eased gently downwards and this exercise will be repeated four or five times.

A Course of Treatment

Although one treatment may be of benefit, it is generally advisable for a course of treatment to be followed and the optimum length for this will depend greatly on the conditions present and the receptiveness of the patient to treatment. Treatment at weekly intervals is usually advised as this gives the body a chance to begin its self-repairing work in between treatments. It also means that if there are any reactions to treatment, then these have a chance to settle down before further treatment is given. There are some occasions when treatment can be given twice a week and this can be particularly helpful for such conditions as a bad back where the trouble might have arisen due to a direct injury, such as a pulled muscle. In such cases, when the body is working quite well in other respects, there is less risk of overworking the systems or causing strong healing reactions.

It is usually recommended that a person has an initial course of at least three treatments. By the time three treatments have been given, some response to the treatment should have occurred. They may feel completely better, have seen an improvement in their condition or may just feel a general change for the better in themselves. If after three treatments, no difference in any way whatsoever has been experienced, then it may be that in this particular instance reflexology treatment is not going to help them.

More often than not, more than three treatments will be required and the average length of a course of treatment is between six to eight treatments, although obviously this is variable. Often, if treatment has been helpful, a person may decide to continue the treatment but leave longer intervals between the treatments possibly extending the gap to two, then three or more weeks. Then, as a general form of 'body maintenance', treatment could be given at, for example, monthly or two-monthly intervals. This will, of course, depend entirely on the individual, the nature of their complaint and how they have responded to the reflexology treatment they have had. It may even be that a person decides to have treatment once a week for an extended period and this is quite acceptable. Certainly regular treatment is a good thing for nearly everyone.

Self-treatment

For self-treatment to the feet, the patient should sit with the knee bent to enable the sole of the foot to be viewed. In this position it should be possible to reach all the reflex points, though the foot will need to be turned to work the outer side of the foot. Some people, however, find reaching the feet to treat them rather difficult and then the hands are often the more sensible area to work on for self-treatment since they are more easily reached. For either form of self-treatment, the patient should sit as comfortably as possible in a quiet environment and follow the recommended order of treatment.

Self-treatment can be most effective, particularly for relieving symptoms by working on just certain important reflexes rather than giving a full treatment. For example, being able to work on the reflexes to the head to relieve a headache is very useful. However, a full treatment of all the reflex points is best and will have longer lasting effects.

Although self-treatment is better than no treatment and is a way to maintain good health, to receive treatment from another person is preferable, particularly when a certain disorder is known to be present, and also because it is more relaxing. To most people this latter factor is a most important part of the treatment and it is not so easy to achieve with self-treatment. Self-treatment, however, is often the way in which people have been introduced to reflexology. They may have read an article or a book on the subject and experimented by massaging areas on their own feet or hands. On seeing the results, they realize the great potential of reflexology and a visit to a professional practitioner for a more thorough treatment follows.

5 Reactions to Treatment and When Not to Treat

Reactions to Treatment

One of the main reasons for people seeking complementary therapies is a growing awareness that the drugs prescribed by orthodox doctors can, in many cases, have unpleasant side-effects and result in other problems developing. Although reflexology does not produce these sorts of side-effects, it is possible that reactions to treatment may occur. These reactions are often referred to as healing reactions as they are a means by which the body clears toxins from the system in order for the body to be able to heal itself. They will appear mainly as a result of increased activity of the body's eliminatory systems, such as the lungs, the kidneys, the intestines and the skin that can occur following reflexology treatment. Provided that treatment is given carefully, these reactions should not be so strong as to cause any inconvenience to the patient and they should be regarded as a good sign, that the body is attempting to put itself right. Usually these reactions will last no more than 24 to 48 hours.

The following are examples of the types of reactions that can occur:

- with the respiratory system, if there is congestion in the sinuses, the patient may show symptoms of a cold and if there is congestions in the lungs, the patient may show symptoms of a cough and these are both ways in which the body clears congested excess mucus from the system
- with the kidneys, it is quite common that, following

treatment, patients find that they need to pass urine more frequently and that the urine may have a different colour and odour than usual

- where there is congestion in the digestive system, a patient may find that the bowels are emptied more frequently and more flatulence may occur
- with a skin condition, a skin rash may become worse after treatment before improving and this is particularly the case if suppressive ointments have previously been used for the skin condition
- with an arthritic condition, sometimes more pain is experienced in the affected joint for up to 24 hours after treatment before the pain lessens
- in women there may be increased vaginal secretion, which may be slightly acidic and uncomfortable
- with stomach problems, there may be a feeling of nausea after treatment, so it is best that food is not eaten just before treatment, particularly when there are digestive problems
- sometimes patients experience a headache or even a migraine after treatment
- it is quite common for people to feel very tired after treatment and this tiredness should not be fought as it is the body's way of saying that it needs rest for healing to take place
- some people may feel full of energy after treatment
- a common reaction to treatment is that a patient feels relaxed and this may be accompanied by a sense of well-being
- other possible reactions include nosebleeds, sneezing, yawning and I have even had a patient who reported that their fingers became double-jointed after treatment!

When Not to Treat

There are very few instances when treatment is not appropriate at all, but there are many instances when treatment has to be given with extra care and so should be given by a qualified practitioner. Treatment should not be given in the following instances:

- to a person who has an infectious disease

- to a person with a fever or very high temperature
- to a person who has a deep vein thrombosis or a thrombophlebitis
- to a person who has just had replacement surgery
- to a person with severe osteoporosis (decalcification of the bones), particularly if the feet and hands are affected
- to a woman during an unstable or risk pregnancy.

Treatment may be given but extra care must be taken if a patient:

- has a heart condition
- is pregnant (particularly if there is high risk of miscarriage)
- is epileptic (in some instances reflexology may cause an epileptic to have a fit)
- is diabetic (particularly if the patient is on medication as the dosage required may need to be adjusted as a result of reflexology treatment)
- is on medication (it may be necessary for medication to be adjusted as the reflexology treatment becomes effective, for example in cases of high blood pressure or underactivity or overactivity of the thyroid gland).

In cases where the medication taken is painkillers, tranquillizers or antidepressants, this can sometimes rather numb the reflexes. Therefore, although a patient may not report feeling any tenderness when the reflexes are worked on, the treatment can still be taking effect so care has to be taken in these instances in order not to overwork by using too much pressure to try to produce a tangible response for the patient from the tender reflexes.

It is always important to give treatment carefully, but this is particularly so at the start of a course of treatment as some people do react very strongly to the therapy. Overworking is the thing to avoid. By overworking, I mean working too heavily on the reflex points or working on them too frequently or for too long. It has already been stated that the pressure used for the massage should be one that it is comfortable to apply, without involving any effort. Normally a treatment session will last no longer than an hour and the treatment will be given at weekly intervals to allow the body a chance to adjust in response to the treatment and to allow any healing reactions that may occur a chance to subside. It must be remembered that most conditions do not suddenly develop, but have been building up over a period of time, so it is unrealistic to expect instant improvement. Sometimes an immediate improvement is achieved, but this should be followed up by a couple of further treatments to ensure that the improvement is a lasting one. As a very general rule, a course of six to eight reflexology treatments will be required to return the body to balance and this improvement will be permanent, but obviously, further problems might well develop in the future as the many factors of life-style, diet and so on have their effects.

Apart from the conditions specifically mentioned above, it is possible to give reflexology treatment to people suffering from most other conditions. Even where very serious disorders are present, treatment may be given to help alleviate pain, improve the circulation of the blood and the functioning of the eliminatory systems in order to help clear unwanted toxins from the body. It may also aid sleep, relaxation and well-being, which are powerful positive effects in themselves.

6 *The Female Reproductive System and Other Hormonal Glands*

The Female Reproductive System

Before looking at some of the common conditions that specifically affect women, a brief look at the female reproductive system and other hormonal (endocrine) glands will help to provide some explanation as to why some of the problems affecting these systems occur.

The female reproductive system consists of the internal organs lying in the pelvic cavity and the external genitalia. The internal organs are the two ovaries, the two Fallopian (uterine) tubes, the uterus and the vagina; the external genitalia, collectively known as the vulva, are the labia majora, labia minora, clitoris, vestibule, hymen and greater vestibular glands. The breasts (mammary glands) are accessory glands of the female reproductive system.

The Ovaries These are the female sex glands and lie on the lateral walls of the pelvis.

Within each ovary are areas known as the ovarian follicles and each of these contains an ovum, the female reproductive cell which if fertilized by the sperm, the male reproductive cell, will result in pregnancy.

After puberty, during each menstrual cycle until the menopause, one ovarian follicle ruptures and releases its ovum.

The Fallopian Tubes	These extend from the sides of the uterus and pass upwards and outwards to end near each ovary. At the end of each Fallopian tube are finger-like projections that wrap themselves around the ovary.

The purpose of the Fallopian tubes is to convey the ovum from the ovary to the uterus. Fertilization of the ovum takes place within the Fallopian tubes and then it (called the zygote) passes to the uterus.

The Uterus   It is a hollow, pear-shaped organ lying in the pelvic cavity between the bladder and the rectum and it is positioned so that it leans slightly forwards, almost at right angles to the vagina. It can be divided into three parts: the fundus, the body and the cervix.

After puberty, the uterus goes through a cycle of changes known as the menstrual cycle. These prepare it to receive, nourish and protect a fertilized ovum. Each cycle lasts approximately 26 to 30 days and, if fertilization does not occur, the cycle ends with a short period of bleeding known as menstruation.

The Vagina   It connects the internal organs of the female reproductive system with the external genitalia.

Between puberty and the menopause, it provides an acid environment, due to the presence of acid secreting bacteria, to help prevent the growth of microbes that might infect the internal organs.

The Menstrual Cycle

At puberty, the pituitary gland in the brain produces the gonadotrophic hormones follicle stimulating hormone (FSH) and luteinizing hormone (LH) that stimulate the ovaries, so starting the menstrual cycle. At this time the secondary sexual characteristics develop, such as the breasts growing, body hair appearing and the body taking on a more womanly shape. Changes in the hormonal levels associated with puberty start in girls, on average, from the ages of 6 to 8 years but the more noticeable effects just mentioned occur from 10 to 12 years.

It can take two to three years, however, for a normal menstrual cycle to be established.

During the menstrual cycle, a series of changes take place in the walls of the ovaries and uterus in response to the changes in the levels of hormones in the blood. The main hormones involved are oestrogen and progesterone. There are three phases to the menstrual cycle.

First, the FSH from the pituitary promotes the development of an ovarian follicle in the ovaries and the secretion of oestrogen by the follicle. The oestrogen affects the uterus and particularly the endometrium, which is the layer of cells lining the uterus that are prepared to receive a fertilized ovum. This phase ends when ovulation occurs and oestrogen production stops.

Second, directly after ovulation, the cells lining the ovarian follicle are stimulated by LH and the corpus luteum develops in the ovarian follicle, producing progesterone. The progesterone acts on the endometrium of the uterus to cause secretion of increased amounts of a watery mucus and has a similar effect on the glands of the uterine tubes and the cervical glands, which affect the vagina.

Third, if fertilization does not occur, there is a reduction in the activity of the pituitary gland and in the production of LH due to the high progesterone level. The reduction of LH causes the corpus luteum in the ovary to degenerate and, therefore, progesterone production decreases. About 14 days after ovulation, the lining of the uterus will break down and the phase of menstruation begins, which is when the cells of the endometrium, along with the unfertilized ovum and blood, are passed through the vagina.

Once the progesterone level drops to a certain level, FSH will cause the development of another ovarian follicle and this cycle will be repeated.

Pregnancy

If fertilization occurs, then the endometrium will not break down, there will be no menstrual flow and the fertilized ovum will travel down the Fallopian tube to be implanted in the wall of the uterus. The corpus luteum will continue to secrete progesterone for about three to four months, thus inhibiting the development of further ovarian follicles.

During these months, the placenta develops and produces oestrogen, progesterone and gonadotrophins and it is through the placenta that the foetus can obtain nutrients, oxygen, antibodies and remove carbon dioxide and other waste products.

The Menopause

The menopause occurs between the ages of 45 to 55 years and marks the end of a woman's child-bearing years. It can occur quite suddenly or take place over a period of years. At this time there are changes in the concentration of the sex hormones with the ovaries becoming less responsive to the FSH and LH from the pituitary, so ovulation and menstruation become irregular and eventually cease. The menopause can be accompanied by many side-effects due to the drop in hormone levels.

Hormonal Glands

As mentioned previously, other hormonal glands influence the activity of the reproductive glands and these glands are often important in helping to balance the hormone levels in the body and correct reproductive gland problems. We shall therefore take a brief look at these other hormonal glands.

The Pituitary Gland

The pituitary gland is about the size of a pea and is found in the brain, lying in the pituitary fossa at the base of the skull. The hypothalamus also lies in the base of the brain and is connected to the pituitary gland by the pituitary stalk. Together the pituitary and the hypothalamus regulate the activity of most of the other endocrine glands of the body.

The pituitary produces many different hormones and therefore is involved in many different functions in the body. The hypothalamus produces hormones that control the secretions of nearly all the pituitary hormones. The anterior part of the pituitary produces:

- growth hormone (GH), which controls development before puberty and promotes protein synthesis in growth and repair of tissues
- thyroid stimulating hormone (TSH), which stimulates growth and activity of the thyroid gland
- adrenocorticotrophic hormone (ACTH), which stimulates the adrenal cortex to produce the hormone cortisol
- prolactin, which activates the secretion of milk by the breast for lactation
- gonadotrophic hormones, follicle stimulating hormone (FSH) and luteinizing hormone (LH), which affect the development of the ovarian follicle and therefore influence the levels of oestrogen and progesterone in the body.

The posterior part of the pituitary produces:

- oxytocin, which promotes the contraction of the uterine muscles and the contraction of the cells of the breast during breastfeeding
- antidiuretic hormone (ADH), vasopressin, which controls water reabsorption in the kidneys.

The Thyroid Gland

The thyroid gland is situated in the front of the lower part of the neck and consists of two lobes connected by a narrow portion called the isthmus, which lies in front of the windpipe (trachea). It produces the hormones thyroxine (T3) and triiodothyronine (T4), which are important for promoting growth and differentiation of tissues and controlling the basal metabolic rate of the body (the rate at which the oxidative reactions take place and therefore body heat). The thyroid also produces a hormone called calcitonin, which reduces the level of calcium in the blood. This is working in opposition to the parathyroid hormone from the parathyroid glands so together these two hormones regulate the level of calcium in the blood within narrow limits.

The Adrenal Glands

There are two adrenal glands in the body, one situated on top of each kidney, just above waist level. They can be divided into an outer region, known as the adrenal cortex, and an inner region, known as the adrenal medulla.

The adrenal medulla produces the hormones adrenalin and noradrenalin, which help the body cope with adverse environmental conditions. Adrenalin is often known as the 'fear, fight and flight' hormone as it prepares the body to cope with these situations. Noradrenalin helps to maintain the blood pressure.

The adrenal cortex produces:

- mineralcorticoids (aldosterone), which act on the kidneys to adjust the reabsorption of sodium
- glucocorticoids (cortisol - hydrocortisone, corticosterone), which regulate carbohydrate metabolism, can cause the deposition of fat and can depress the body's inflammatory and allergic reactions
- sex hormones (androgens), but these have only a minor effect compared to those produced by the reproductive glands.

The Actions of Hormones

Hormones are often present in precursor forms and show a structural change before presenting as the active form of the hormone. One example of this is a hormone secreted by the hypothalamus that can split to eventually form ACTH (produced by the pituitary and mentioned above) and melanotrophin stimulating hormone (MSH), which influences the formation of melanin, the pigment in the skin. This latter hormone can then further divide to form further substances, including endorphins. The endorphins found in the brain influence such things as:

- the modification of and perception of pain
- regulation of body temperature
- inhibition of the pituitary hormones LH, FSH, ACTH, TSH, vasopressin and oxytocin
- stimulation of the pituitary hormones GH and prolactin.

It is thought that endorphins may play a role in amenorrhoea (absence of menstrual flow), particularly that induced by exercising a great deal, and also, possibly, in premenstrual syndrome.

It is thus apparent that there is a close link between many of the parts of the hormonal system and that a feedback system operates between the pituitary gland and the thyroid, adrenal and reproductive glands. It is, therefore, quite likely that if one part is not working correctly that other parts may also be involved. Reflexology treatment can be beneficial in the treatment of conditions involving hormonal imbalances as it is able to work on all of the different glands at the same treatment and thus restore the balance between them.

7 Conditions Specific to Women That Respond to Reflexology Treatment

Because the level of hormones in the blood varies throughout the menstrual cycle and the fact that the hormonal system is very easily upset by many factors, including stress and tension, it is hardly surprising that many women experience problems associated with their reproductive system. Many of these problems will respond well to reflexology treatment as the hormonal levels can be returned to balance and the person becomes more relaxed.

The conditions described below are some of the more common problems that women may suffer from. The possible causes of the conditions are mentioned and the approach to treatment is discussed. For each condition the relevant reflexes are listed and some of these are more important to the treatment than others because they are *directly* involved with the problem (direct reflexes - DR) or because they are *associated* with the problem (associated reflexes - AR) and both types may be beneficial in relieving the cause of the problem or the symptoms that may be present.

It should be remembered that in all cases, the best results will be obtained if a full reflexology treatment is given, thereby treating the *whole* body, but the important reflexes mentioned will be those that are likely to require extra attention in order to overcome the particular problem.

Figures 7.1, 7.2, 7.3 and 7.4 show the positions of the reflexes that are the most important in the treatment of problems affecting the female reproductive system.

56 ∾

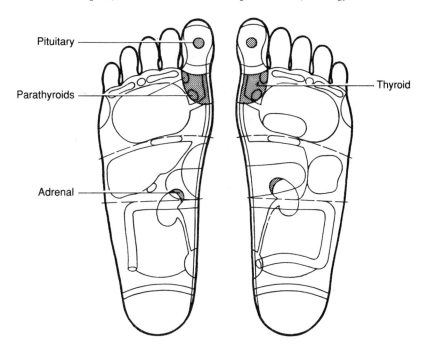

Figure 7.1 *Chart of the soles of the feet showing the reflexes for parts of the hormonal system*

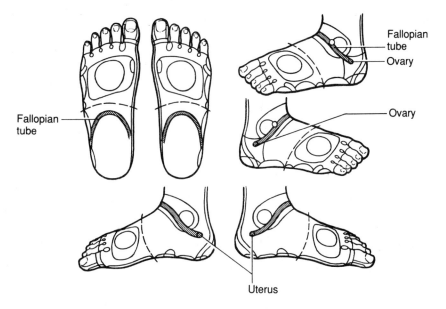

Figure 7.2 *Chart of the tops and sides of the feet showing the reflexes for the female reproductive system*

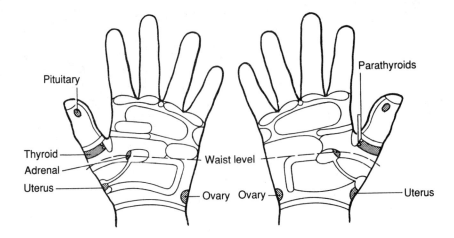

Figure 7.3 *Chart of the palms of the hands showing the reflexes for parts of the hormonal and female reproductive systems*

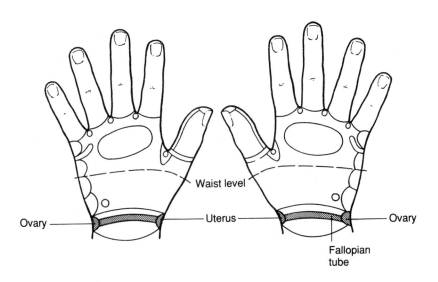

Figure 7.4 *Chart of the backs of the hands showing the reflexes for the female reproductive system*

Menstrual Problems

Amenorrhoea

The condition of amenorrhoea is the absence of menstruation, either when no menstruation has occurred by the age of 16 or when there is an absence of menstruation for a period of about 6 months.

The possibility of the woman being pregnant must first be discounted when there is an absence of menstruation and, in later years, the start of the menopause. Other possible causes can include genetic abnormalities or hormonal imbalances and amenorrhoea can sometimes also occur when a woman stops taking the contraceptive pill. The hormonal imbalances may involve the hypothalamus, the pituitary, the thyroid, the ovaries or the adrenal glands. It is the hypothalamus that is involvedwhen amenorrhoea is associated with weight loss or anorexia nervosa or results from excessive exercise or stress. The pituitary is involved where there is a more serious cause and the thyroid or adrenal glands may be involved where there is either overactivity or underactivity of these glands. Cysts in the ovaries can be another possible cause.

DR: uterus.
AR: ovaries, pituitary, thyroid, adrenals, solar plexus (for relaxation), stomach, small and large intestine (if associated with eating disorder).

Dysmenorrhoea

The condition of dysmenorrhoea is pain relating to menstruation and can occur when the periods first start or after some years of pain-free periods. The pain can start with the onset of menstruation or a few days before menstruation and is more severe for the first few days of a period, with pain being experienced in the abdomen and possibly feelings of a bloated abdomen, together with nausea, migraines and joint pains. It will be associated with a problem in the uterus, which may be endometriosis (see page 64), a polyp or fibroid or may be caused by the presence of an intra-uterine contraceptive device (IUCD).

DR: uterus.
AR: abdominal areas (to alleviate pain), top of head, side of head, eyes (for migraines), stomach (for nausea), joint reflexes (if joint pain), solar plexus (for relaxation).

Irregular Periods (Metrorrhagia)

Irregular periods (or metrorrhagia) means that menstruation does not follow a regular pattern. Individuals will normally show different patterns in their menstrual cycles - differences in the length of the cycle, differences in the amount of bleeding at the time of menstruation and differences in the length of time that menstruation lasts - but, if a regular pattern for that individual is not established then that person's periods are irregular. This is usually due to a hormone imbalance, which is often associated with stress and tension.

DR: ovaries, Fallopian tubes, uterus, pituitary.
AR: thyroid, adrenals, solar plexus (for relaxation).

Menorrhagia

The condition of menorrhagia is that of excessive menstrual loss and may be associated with a problem involving the uterus, such as fibroids, polyps, infection, pelvic inflammatory disease, endometritis (see page 64), endometriosis (see page 64) or the presence of an IUCD. Other possible causes can include sterilization, depression and hormonal imbalances of the ovaries or thyroid.

DR: uterus.
AR: ovaries, pituitary, thyroid, pelvic lymphatics (if infection is present).

Premenstrual Syndrome (PMS)

In premenstrual syndrome there is an exaggeration of the normal physiological and psychological differences in well-being that can occur for a few days before menstruation. In severe cases, the problems may be present for as many as ten days prior to menstruation and the symptoms can include any, or even all, of the following: anxiety, irritability, lack of concentration, depression, changes in appetite, fatigue, headaches, abdominal pains, backache, tenderness in the breasts, fluid retention, constipation and skin problems such as spots, boils or acne on the face.

DR: ovaries, Fallopian tubes, uterus, pituitary.
AR: thyroid, adrenals, head and brain (if headaches), spine (if backache), abdomen (if abdominal pains), breasts (if breast tenderness), bladder, kidneys (if fluid retention), small and large intestines (if constipation), face (if skin problems), solar plexus (for relaxation).

Infertility

Infertility is the state of being unable to conceive after one year of unprotected intercourse and the term may be used to refer to a state of having never conceived or that of having difficulty in conceiving again after having previously conceived.

Possible causes may include a failure to ovulate, a blockage in the Fallopian tubes, an imbalance in the pH of the cervical mucus or a problem involving the sperm from the male, such as a low sperm count. A failure to ovulate may involve problems with the hormonal system, such as the hypothalamus, pituitary, thyroid, adrenals or ovaries. If the cause of infertility has not been established, then it is best for both partners to receive treatment so as not to place the responsibility on one or other.

DR: ovaries, Fallopian tubes, uterus.
AR: pituitary, thyroid, adrenals, solar plexus (for relaxation).

Pregnancy

Although pregnancy is not a illness, it can cause problems which can distress the pregnant woman. These can include sickness and nausea, constipation, increased frequency of passing urine, backache and sciatica. Reflexology can be used to keep a woman healthy during pregnancy and the treatment should also help with the development of a healthy baby.

It must be stressed that *great care must be taken with the treatment of a woman who is pregnant*, particularly if there is a history of miscarriage or during a first pregnancy. It would be unwise for self-treatment to be given during pregnancy and the help of a qualified practitioner should be sought who will be able to advise whether or not reflexology treatment is appropriate in a particular case.

DR: stomach (for nausea), intestines (for constipation), bladder, ureter tubes, kidneys (for frequency of passing urine), lower spine (for pain and sciatica), sciatic reflexes (for sciatica).
AR: ovaries, uterus, pituitary, breasts.

Childbirth

Many midwives now use reflexology to help at the time of childbirth, particularly to help with pain or if birth is delayed or uterine contractions are weak.

DR: uterus.
AR: pituitary, lower spine (for back pain), solar plexus (for relaxation).

Postnatal Symptoms

A woman may experience postnatal symptoms as the hormone levels in the body readjust and the body itself readjusts after the months of pregnancy.

Possible symptoms may include tiredness, depression, urinary infections, discomfort in the breasts or difficulty with breastfeeding.

DR: ovaries, uterus, pituitary.
AR: head and brain areas (for depression), bladder, ureter tubes, kidneys, pelvic lymphatics (if urinary infections), breasts, lymph nodes of axilla (if breast discomfort or difficulty with breastfeeding).

Menopausal Problems

At the time of the menopause, the periods will become irregular and will vary from heavy to scanty ones.

Problems associated with the menopause can include depression, insomnia, headaches, failing memory, indigestion, flatulence, constipation, increased frequency of passing urine, thinning of skin, atrophy of the breasts, loss of interest in sex, hot flushes and osteoporosis (brittle bones). The problems are due to the reduced level of oestrogen present in the body.

DR: ovaries, uterus, pituitary.
AR: head and brain areas (for depression, headaches, insomnia), stomach (for indigestion), intestines (for constipation and flatulence), bladder, ureter tubes, kidneys (for increased frequency of passing urine), breasts (for breast problems), thyroid and parathyroids (to help restore calcium balance), solar plexus (for relaxation).

Breast Lumps

Breast lumps may be due to the presence of a cyst, a tumour (harmless or cancerous) or mastitis (see page 65).

It is important that if a woman discovers a lump in the breast that professional advice be sought in case it proves to be cancerous.

DR: breasts.
AR: lymph nodes of axilla.

Cervicitis

Cervicitis is the inflammation of the cervix, usually due to infection. It may be associated with a high oestrogen level in the blood or oversecretion of the glands in the cervix. There may be symptoms of pain in the lower back, pelvis and legs, increased frequency of passing urine, painful periods and an increased vaginal discharge (leukorrhoea).

DR: uterus.
AR: ovaries, Fallopian tubes, pituitary, adrenals, pelvic lymphatics (for infection), lower spine (for backache), hip and knee (for leg pains), bladder, ureter tube, kidneys (for increased frequency of passing urine).

Endometritis

The condition of endometritis is the inflammation of the endometrium (the tissue lining the uterus) and this may be caused by infection or pelvic inflammatory disease.

Symptoms present may include pain in the centre of the lower pelvis, increased frequency of passing urine with burning (similar to that experienced by cystitis sufferers) and an increased vaginal secretion. It can lead to adhesions, salpingitis (see page 66), obstruction of the Fallopian tubes and infertility if untreated.

DR: uterus.
AR: Fallopian tubes, ovaries, pelvic lymphatics (if infection present).

Endometriosis

In the condition of endometriosis, endometrium tissue is found in abnormal sites in the body, most commonly on the ovaries, Fallopian tubes and pelvic structures. This tissue reacts to the monthly variation in hormones in a similar way to the way in which it does in the uterus, causing menstrual-like bleeding. Unlike the menstrual flow, the blood cannot escape, causing pain and inflammation or blood-filled cysts. There may be symptoms of intermittent pain due to the swelling caused and also the bleeding may lead to the formation of fibrous scar tissue as the body tries to heal itself and, over time, ovarian endometriosis can build into pelvic adhesions when nearby organs become stuck together - ovary to bowel.

DR: ovaries, Fallopian tubes, pelvis (possible sites of problem).
AR: intestines (if adhesions in this area).

Fibroids

Fibroids are fairly common, harmless growths found in the uterus, but they can lead to increased bleeding at menstruation and may also be accompanied by irregular bleeding, abdominal and pelvic pain or increased frequency of passing water. Often fibroids regress after the menopause.

DR: uterus.
AR: ovaries, Fallopian tubes, pituitary, bladder (if increased frequency of passing urine), abdominal areas (if pain).

Mastitis

With mastitis there is inflammation of the breasts with pain and swelling (particularly before a period) and, occasionally, discharge from the nipple. The breasts may also feel lumpy. The condition is more common among women nearing the menopause who have not been pregnant or have not breastfed. Chronic mastitis is also known as fibrocystic disease or fibroadenosis.

DR: breasts.
AR: adrenals (for inflammation), lymph nodes of axilla (if infection is present), pituitary (for hormone balance).

Ovarian Cysts

In the majority of women up to the time of the menopause, ovarian cysts will be benign. They may, however, cause pain in the abdomen, disorders of the digestive tract and increased frequency of passing urine.

DR: ovaries.
AR: Fallopian tubes, uterus, intestines (if digestive problems), bladder (if increased frequency of passing urine), abdominal areas (if pain).

Salpingitis

With salpingitis there is inflammation of the Fallopian tubes with the infection usually spreading from the uterus. The infection can then spread to the ovaries and there may be problems with blocked Fallopian tubes, infertility and adhesions in the pelvis.

DR: Fallopian tubes.
AR: ovaries, uterus, pelvic lymphatics (for infection), adrenals (for inflammation).

Thrush

Candida albicans is a fungus that consists of yeast-like cells that are normally present in humans in the mouth, throat, gut, skin and vagina. When the body's defence systems are low, however, this can then become pathogenic and give rise to conditions such as thrush.

With thrush there may be symptoms of irritation, burning and itching of the vulva and the entrance to the vagina which may appear red, a white, yeast-smelling discharge and increased frequency of passing urine together with a burning sensation.

DR: uterus (to include vagina).
AR: lymphatics, especially pelvic lymphatics (for infection), spleen (for body's defence system), adrenals (for inflammation and stress).

Vaginitis

Vaginitis is inflammation of the vagina, causing vaginal pain and irritation.

DR: uterus (including reflex for vagina).
AR: pelvic lymphatics (for infection), adrenals (for inflammation).

Some Effects of Treatment

As a result of reflexology treatment, it is sometimes found that the menstrual cycle alters in some way, such as periods occurring earlier or there being a slightly heavier blood loss. However, these reactions should be only temporary if a course of treatment is followed and a regular pattern will develop.

For women taking the contraceptive pill, there is no evidence to suggest that reflexology treatment will interfere with the effectiveness of this. If an IUCD is fitted, in some instances this may be detected during reflexology treatment as being a 'foreign' item in the body and the device, particularly if it is not fitted well, may move. Although this is not a common reaction, it is one to be aware of.

Many women nowadays receive hormone replacement therapy (HRT) to counteract the effects on the body that can occur after the menopause as a result of the body ceasing to produce these hormones itself. This form of treatment supplies additional oestrogen and sometimes also progesterone to the body and is considered helpful in preventing such problems as osteoporosis, which is when the bones become brittle and more likely to fracture. Although it is quite safe for a person receiving HRT to have reflexology treatment, it is unlikely that reflexology will be effective in helping to resolve the hormonal imbalance problem while the patient is receiving HRT. Therefore, it is best that treatment for a menopausal problem is given when the patient is *not* receiving HRT. For problems other than those for which the HRT is being given, however, reflexology treatment can be very helpful.

8 General Conditions That Respond to Reflexology Treatment

The following conditions are ones that do not affect only women but which often occur in both sexes. After a brief discussion of the condition, the direct (DR) and associated (AR) reflexes that will be helpful in treating the condition are given and, as in the last chapters, these are the reflexes that may require extra attention during a reflexology treatment of the whole body.

Allergies

An allergy is oversensitivity to a substance either eaten, inhaled or touched. This may manifest itself as a skin rash (nettlerash, ezcema, dermatitis), hay fever, rhinitis, asthma, headaches, diarrhoea or vomiting. Obviously where possible and where the allergy is known, it is best to simply avoid the offending substances, but reflexology treatment can sometimes help to reduce the sensitivity to them.

DR: dependent on part of body affected, but could include lungs, digestive system, skin, nose, sinuses (see Figures 8.1a and b).
AR: adrenals (for anti-allergy properties), spleen (for allergies), solar plexus (for relaxation) (see Figure 8.1a).

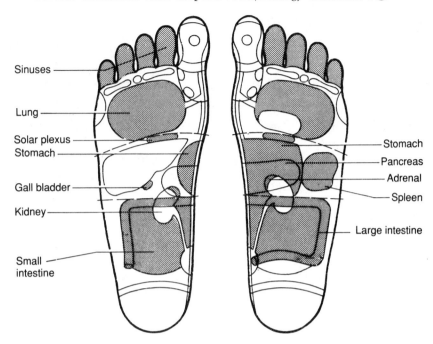

Figure 8.1a *Chart of the soles of the feet showing the reflexes used in treating allergies*

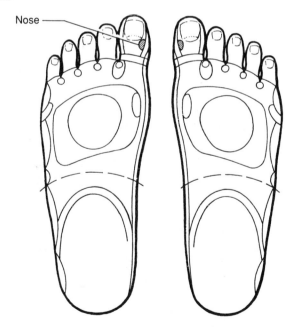

Figure 8.1b *Chart of the tops of the feet showing the reflexes used in treating allergies*

Arthritis

The term arthritis is used to describe inflammation and pain in a joint. There are many different types of arthritis, including osteoarthritis and rheumatoid arthritis, but the approach to treating it with reflexology will be the same whatever type it is.

The effectiveness of the treatment will probably be influenced by the severity of the condition but the prime aim will be to help relieve pain and reduce inflammation, though, in some cases, even greater improvement may be achieved.

DR: joint affected (e.g., spine, hip, knee, shoulder – see Figure 8.2b).
AR: zone-related area (i.e., shoulder for hip, elbow for knee, etc., with massage being applied directly to the zone-related area and to the zone-related reflex), adrenals (for inflammation), solar plexus (for relaxation), thyroid and parathyroids (for calcium balance), small and large intestines (for elimination), kidneys (for elimination), pituitary (for hormone balance) – see Figures 8.2a and b.

Asthma

A patient suffering from asthma experiences bouts of breathlessness due to temporary closure of the smaller airways deep in the lung tissues and this may be accompanied by tightness in the chest or throat and a feeling of suffocation with wheezing breathing. Asthma may be associated with an allergy, stress or a chronic lung condition.

DR: lungs, bronchi (see Figure 8.3).
AR: solar plexus, diaphragm (both for relaxation), adrenals (for allergy, stress), cervical and thoracic spine (for nerve supply to bronchi and lungs), heart (asthma attacks may put added strain on the heart), ileo-caecal valve and intestines (for healthy elimination) – see Figure 8.3.

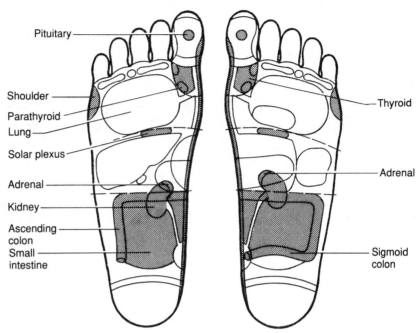

Figure 8.2a *Chart of the soles of the feet showing the reflexes used in treating arthritis*

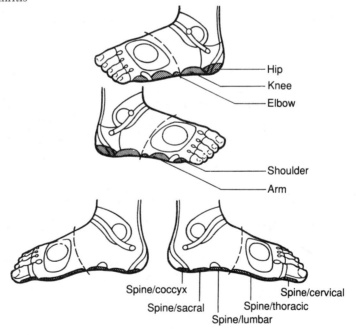

Figure 8.2b *Chart of the sides of the feet showing the reflexes used in treating arthritis*

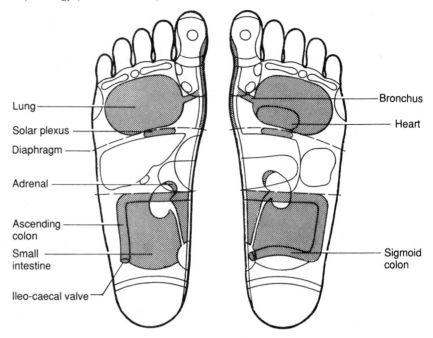

Lung

Solar plexus

Diaphragm

Adrenal

Ascending colon

Small intestine

Ileo-caecal valve

Bronchus

Heart

Sigmoid colon

Figure 8.3a *Chart of the soles of the feet showing the reflexes used in treating asthma*

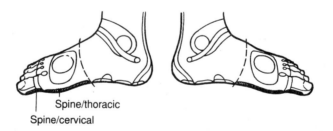

Spine/thoracic

Spine/cervical

Figure 8.3b *Chart of the sides of the feet showing the reflexes used in treating asthma*

Back Pain

Back pain can be caused by many things and is one of the most common ailments. The pain may be associated with a muscle strain or pulled ligament or may involve the actual bony vertebrae of the spine becoming displaced.

Although it is not possible to diagnose the exact cause of the problem using reflexology, the treatment is most effective for many causes of back pain.

DR: spine, neck (see Figures 8.4a and b).
AR: solar plexus (for pain), adrenals (for inflammation), reflexes for areas affected by the back problem (e.g. leg, sciatic nerve, arm) – see Figures 8.4a and b.

Catarrh

Catarrh is inflammation of a mucous membrane with a constant discharge of mucus and most commonly affects the nose. This may result from a cold, dietary factors, an allergy or from a deformity of the nose or sinusitis.

DR: sinuses, nose (see Figures 8.5a and b).
AR: adrenals (for allergy), ileo-caecal valve (often connected with excess mucus conditions), intestines (for elimination), head (for headaches), upper lymph nodes (if infection present) – see Figures 8.5a and b.

Chilblains

Chilblains are dusky red, oval swellings on the fingers or toes that are intensely itchy. They are caused by poor circulation to the extremities with the blood vessels in the skin not responding correctly to a lowering of the skin temperature. They often occur when it is cold and damp.

DR: zone-related areas (i.e., toes if fingers affected or fingers if toes affected).
AR: heart (for circulation), small and large intestines (for

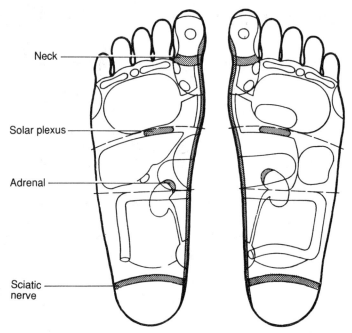

Figure 8.4a *Chart of the soles of the feet showing the reflexes used in treating back pain*

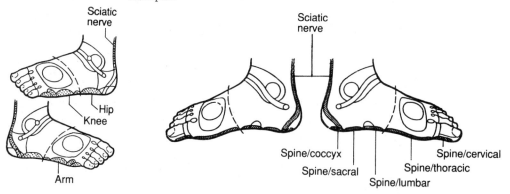

Figure 8.4b *Chart of the sides of the feet showing the reflexes used in treating back pain*

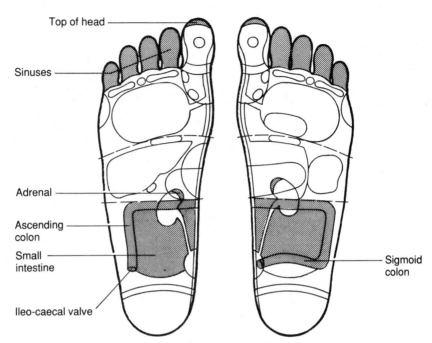

Figure 8.5a *Chart of the soles of the feet showing the reflexes used in treating catarrh*

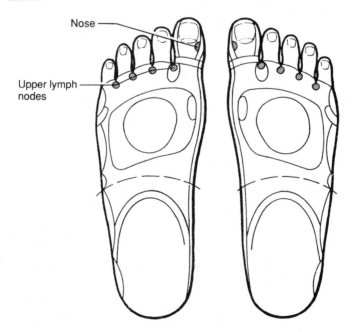

Figure 8.5b *Chart of the tops of the feet showing the reflexes used in treating catarrh*

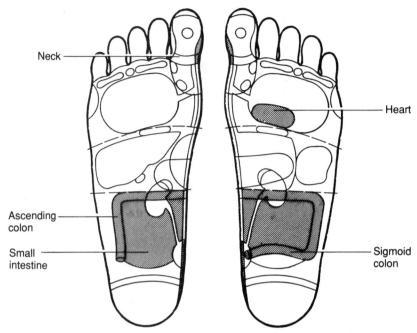

Neck

Heart

Ascending colon

Small intestine

Sigmoid colon

Figure 8.6a *Chart of the soles of the feet showing the reflexes used in treating chilblains*

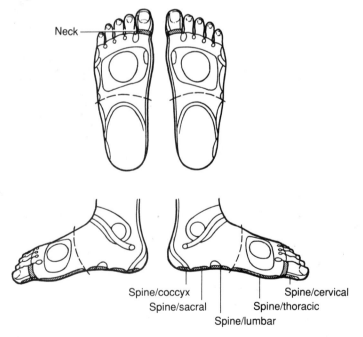

Neck

Spine/coccyx

Spine/sacral

Spine/lumbar

Spine/thoracic

Spine/cervical

Figure 8.6b *Chart of tops and sides of the feet showing the reflexes used in healing chilblains*

healthy elimination), spine (upper region if fingers affected, lower region if toes affected to ensure good working of the nerves to the area) - see Figure 8.6.

Conjunctivitis

Conjunctivitis is an inflammation of the conjunctiva, which is a thin membrane lining the eyelids. It is caused by either infection or an allergy. The eye becomes red and very itchy.

DR: eyes (see Figure 8.7a).
AR: upper lymphatics (for infection), adrenals (for allergy), kidneys (zone-related to eyes and often helpful for treating eye problems) - see Figures 8.7a and b.

Constipation

Constipation is sluggish, irregular emptying of the bowels. This may be caused by dietary factors such as a lack of roughage in the diet or poor muscle tone in the bowel. Persistent constipation can lead to other conditions so it is important that the problem is corrected.

DR: large intestine (particularly hepatic, splenic and sigmoid flexures) - see Figure 8.8.
AR: small intestine, liver, lower spine (for good working of the nerves to the intestines), adrenals (for muscle tone), solar plexus (for relaxation) - see Figure 8.8.

Cystitis

The condition of cystitis is inflammation of the bladder. The symptoms are a burning sensation on passing urine and an increased frequency of so doing. This condition can be a very persistent one and often a person who has suffered from cystitis will have a history of it recurring, particularly when the general health of the body becomes weakened.

DR: bladder (see Figure 8.9a).

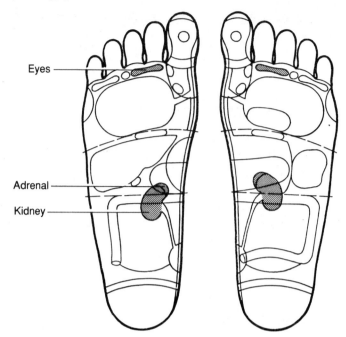

Eyes

Adrenal

Kidney

Figure 8.7a *Chart of the soles of the feet showing the reflexes used in treating conjunctivitis*

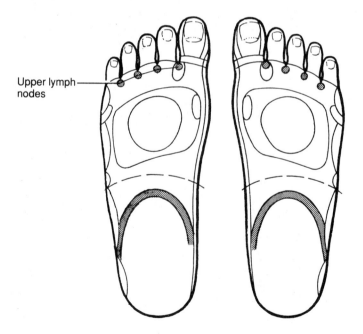

Upper lymph nodes

Figure 8.7b *Chart of the tops of the feet showing the reflexes used in treating conjunctivitis*

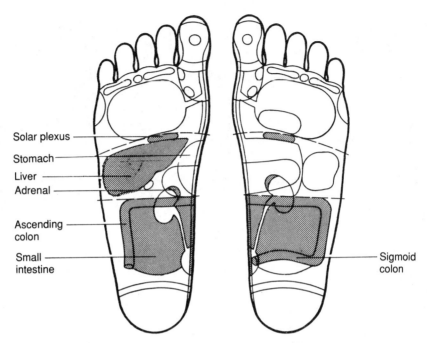

Solar plexus
Stomach
Liver
Adrenal
Ascending colon
Small intestine
Sigmoid colon

Figure 8.8a *Chart of the soles of the feet showing the reflexes used in treating constipation*

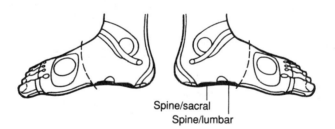

Spine/sacral
Spine/lumbar

Figure 8.8b *Chart of the sides of the feet showing the reflexes used in treating constipation*

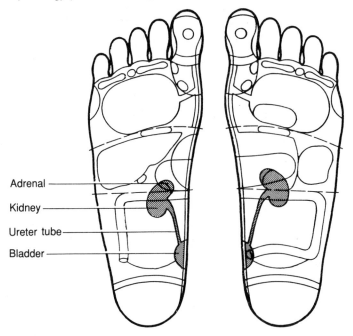

Figure 8.9a *Chart of the soles of the feet showing the reflexes used in treating cystitis*

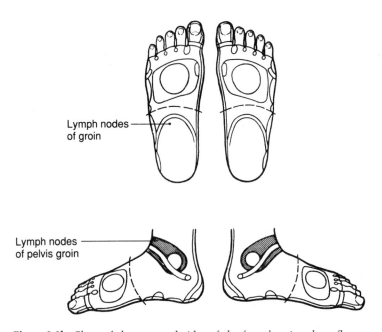

Figure 8.9b *Chart of the tops and sides of the feet showing the reflexes used in treating cystitis*

AR: kidneys, ureter tubes (both parts of urinary system), pelvic lymphatics (for infection), adrenals (for inflammation) - see Figures 8.9a and b.

Depression

Most people suffer from mild bouts of depression at times, but these black moods can lift as quickly as they came. However, when depression really takes over a person there seems no hope and in these cases professional help should be sought. In conjunction with professional help, the general relaxing effect of reflexology can be helpful and its balancing effect on all the systems of the body, many of which may be out of balance, such as the hormonal and the digestive systems, can be beneficial. The hour spent individually with a practitioner can also help psychologically as they have an opportunity to talk freely in a relaxing situation.

DR: head/brain (see Figure 8.10).

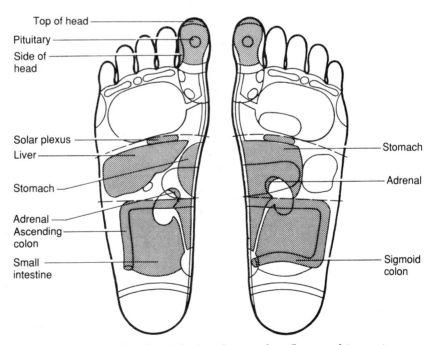

Figure 8.10 *Chart of the soles of the feet showing the reflexes used in treating depression*

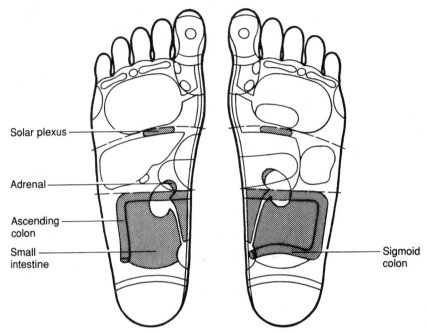

Figure 8.11a *Chart of the soles of the feet showing the reflexes used in treating diarrhoea*

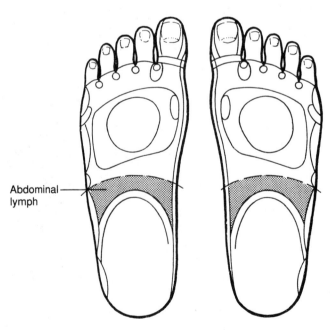

Figure 8.11b *Chart of the tops of the feet showing the reflexes used in treating diarrhoea*

AR: solar plexus (for relaxation), adrenals (for stress), liver (for removal of toxins), pituitary and hormonal system (for any hormonal imbalance), digestive system (for any digestive problems) - see Figure 8.10.

Diarrhoea

With diarrhoea there is increased activity of the bowels and the elimination of watery stools. It is often the body's natural response to a need to clear unwanted material from the body, but, if the condition persists, there is also the problem of the body becoming dehydrated as water reabsorption in the large intestine is reduced.

DR: large intestine (see Figure 8.11a).
AR: small intestine, adrenals (for inflammation and muscle tone), solar plexus (for relaxation, abdominal lymphatics (if infection present) - see Figures 8.11a and b.

Earache

Earache usually results from infection in the outer or middle ear, though it may indicate a more serious problem.

DR: ear (see Figure 8.12a).
AR: Eustachian tube, side of head, solar plexus (for relaxation), upper lymphatics (if infection present) - see Figures 8.12a and b.

Eczema

Eczema is a skin condition in which the skin becomes very dry, red and scaly, accompanied by burning and itching. It may be due to an allergy, dietary factors, hormonal imbalances or stress.

DR: areas of skin affected (e.g., face, elbow, knee) - see Figures 8.13a and b.
AR: adrenals (for anti-allergy and anti-inflammatory properties), solar plexus (for relaxation), kidneys and intestine (to ensure

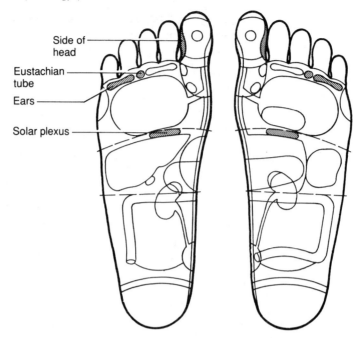

Side of head

Eustachian tube

Ears

Solar plexus

Figure 8.12a *Chart of the soles of the feet showing the reflexes used in treating earache*

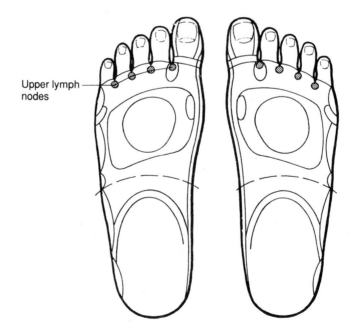

Upper lymph nodes

Figure 8.12b *Chart of the tops of the feet showing the reflexes used in treating earache*

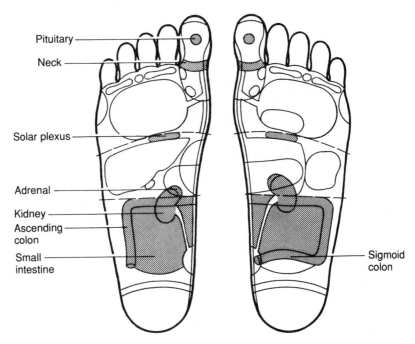

Figure 8.13a *Chart of the soles of the feet showing the reflexes used in treating eczema*

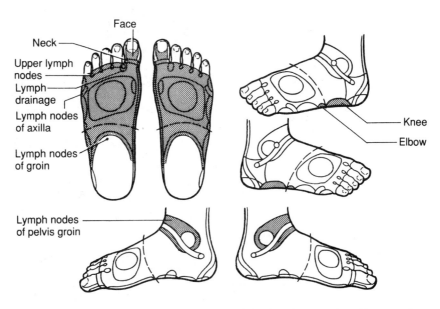

Figure 8.13b *Chart of the tops and sides of the feet showing the reflexes used in treating eczema*

healthy elimination), lymphatics (if infection), pituitary (for hormonal balance) - see Figures 18.13a and b.

Fluid Retention (Oedema)

Fluid retention, or oedema, occurs when excess fluid is retained rather than excreted from the body. Visible swelling of areas of tissues may occur, particularly in the feet and ankles because of the effect of gravity.

This problem quite often occurs during pregnancy, especially later on in the pregnancy, as the hormones cause the body to retain extra fluid. Otherwise it may be associated with disorders of the kidneys, heart, liver or lymphatics. It is also possible for fluid retention to occur in the lungs (pulmonary oedema) and in the eyes (as in glaucoma).

DR: kidneys (see Figure 8.14).
AR: bladder, ureter tubes, pituitary, heart, liver, lymphatics, lungs, eyes (if affected) - see Figure 8.14.

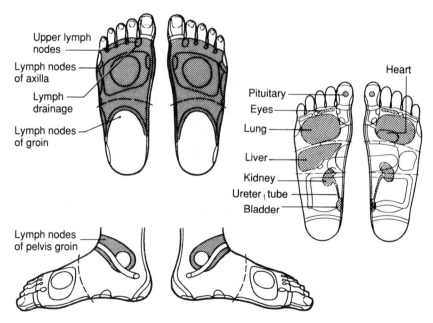

Figure 8.14 *Chart of the tops and soles of the feet showing the reflexes used in treating fluid retention (oedema)*

Haemorrhoids (Piles)

Haemorrhoids, or piles, are varicose veins found around the anus and are often associated with persistent constipation. They can occur externally or internally and will cause pain and bleeding when passing stools.

DR: rectum/anus (see Figure 8.15b).
AR: large intestine, small intestine, heart (for circulation) - see Figure 8.15a.

Hay Fever

Hay fever is an allergy to pollens from grasses and trees.

The symptoms are similar to those of a cold, the person having a streaming and sometimes blocked nose, sneezing and red, watery eyes. The condition occurs seasonally when the pollens that affect the person are present. Similar symptoms occur in the condition of allergic rhinitis where the allergy is to substances other than pollens, such as dust, wool, feathers, animals and foods.

DR: nose, sinuses, eyes (see Figures 8.16a and b)
AR: adrenals (for anti-allergy properties), head, face (for the areas affected) - see Figures 8.16a and b.

High Blood Pressure (Hypertension)

High blood pressure, or hypertension, can lead to symptoms of headaches, dizziness, noises in the ears, breathlessness and chest pains and eyesight problems. There are many possible causes of high blood pressure, but the major factor is often stress and tension.

DR: heart (see Figure 8.17).
AR: solar plexus (for relaxation), adrenals (for stress), head, ears, eyes, lungs, kidneys (for possible symptoms) - see Figure 8.17.

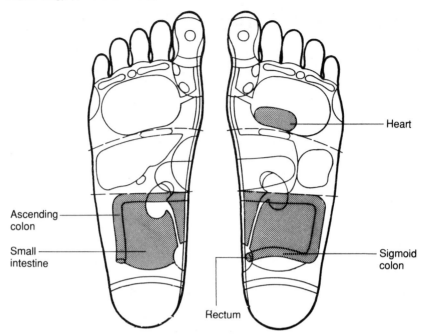

Figure 8.15a *Chart of the soles of the feet showing the reflexes used in treating haemorrhoids (piles)*

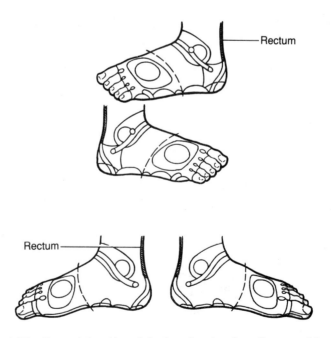

Figure 8.15b *Chart of the sides of the feet showing the reflexes used in treating haemorrhoids (piles)*

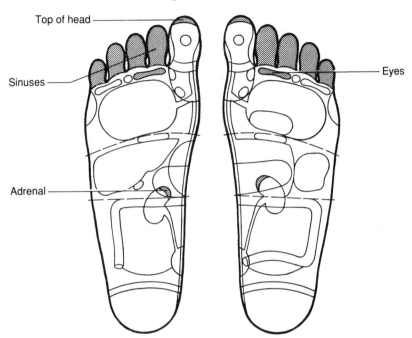

Figure 8.16a *Chart of the soles of the feet showing the reflexes used in treating hay fever*

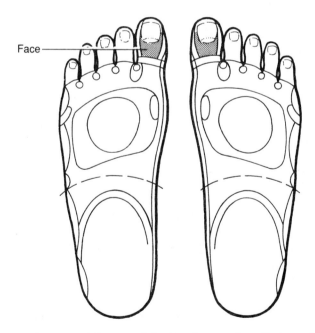

Figure 8.16b *Chart of the tops of the feet showing the reflexes used in treating hay fever*

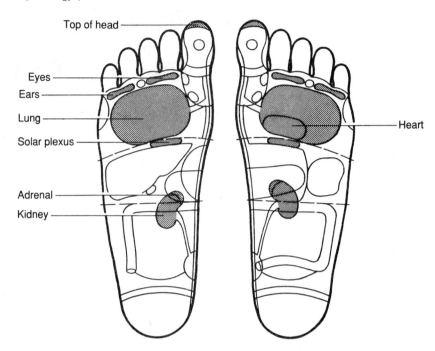

Top of head

Eyes

Ears

Lung

Solar plexus

Adrenal

Kidney

Heart

Figure 8.17 *Chart of the soles of the feet showing the reflexes used in treating high blood pressure (hypertension)*

Insomnia

Insomnia is an inability to get off to sleep, waking early or experiencing disturbed sleep. Most people feel better for a good night's sleep and without sleep become irritable and bad tempered, finding it more difficult to concentrate on tasks. Although insomnia can be caused by physical illness, such as pain, fever, difficulty in breathing and the menopause, a major contributory factor to insomnia is anxiety and worry, including, ironically, worrying that one is not going to sleep. Often the general relaxing and overall balancing effect of reflexology can be of help in this condition.

DR: head/brain (see Figure 8.18).
AR: solar plexus (for relaxation), adrenals (for stress), parts relating to any cause of physical pain (see Figure 8.18) – e.g. lower backache, toothache.

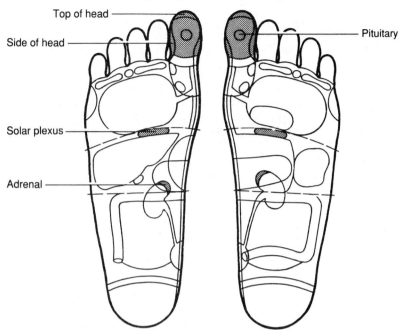

Figure 8.18a *Chart of the soles of the feet showing the reflexes used in treating insomnia*

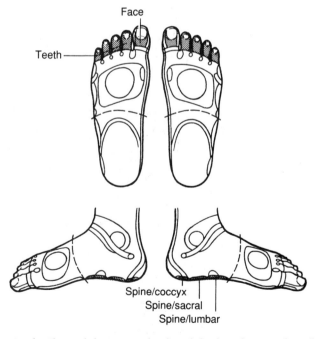

Figure 8.18b *Chart of the tops and sides of the feet showing the reflexes used in treating insomnia*

Irritable Bowel Syndrome

With irritable bowel syndrome (which includes such conditions as mucous colitis and spastic colon) there will be colicky pains with alternating diarrhoea and constipation and an excessive amount of mucus will be present in the stools. There may also be flatulence and bloating of the abdomen.

This condition often afflicts 'nervy' types and can also result from a food allergy. It appears to be more common in women than in men.

DR: large intestine (see Figure 8.19).
AR: small intestine, solar plexus (for relaxation), adrenals (for stress and allergy) – see Figure 8.19.

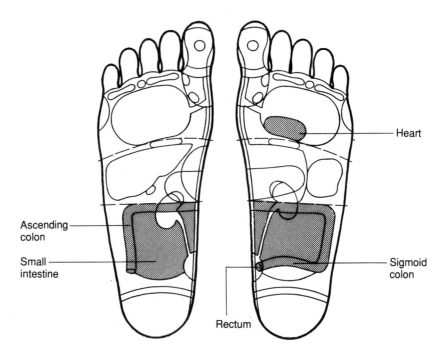

Figure 8.19 *Chart of the soles of the feet showing the reflexes used in treating irritable bowel syndrome*

Migraine

A migraine is a severe form of headache where there may be visual disturbances as well as a very bad headache and possibly nausea and vomiting.

There are many possible causes of this problem, including dietary factors, hormonal changes (associated with the menstrual cycle or menopause), congestion of the sinuses, eye strain, tension in the neck and upper spine and general stress and tension.

DR: head (see Figure 8.20a).
AR: solar plexus (for relaxation), neck, upper spine (for tension), stomach (if nausea), eyes (if eye strain), sinuses (if congested), small and large intestine (if food allergy), pituitary, reproductive areas (if associated with the menstrual cycle or the menopause) – see Figures 8.20a and b.

Myalgic Encephalomyelitis (ME)

ME is sometimes referred to as post-viral fatigue syndrome as the condition results from a viral infection that is followed by extreme fatigue, muscle weakness, depression and digestive disturbances. The symptoms can be very severe and the condition may last for several years. Reflexology treatment can help strengthen the immune system to clear the virus from the system.

DR: lymphatics, spleen (see Figures 8.21a and b).
AR: solar plexus (for relaxation), adrenals (for stress), head/brain (if depression), stomach, intestines (if digestive problems) – see Figure 8.21a.

Neck Pain

Many people suffer from neck pain and this often results from tension. Tightness in the neck muscles can also spread down across the top of the back and to the shoulders.

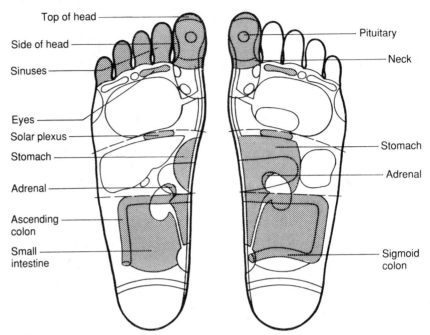

Top of head
Side of head
Sinuses
Eyes
Solar plexus
Stomach
Adrenal
Ascending colon
Small intestine

Pituitary
Neck
Stomach
Adrenal
Sigmoid colon

Figure 8.20a *Chart of the soles of the feet showing the reflexes used in treating migraine*

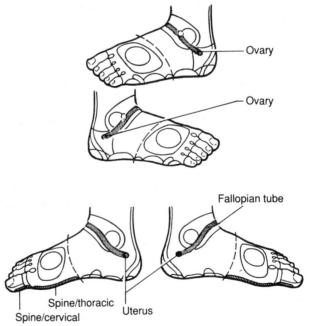

Ovary
Ovary
Fallopian tube
Spine/thoracic
Spine/cervical
Uterus

Figure 8.20b *Chart of the sides of the feet showing the reflexes used in treating migraine*

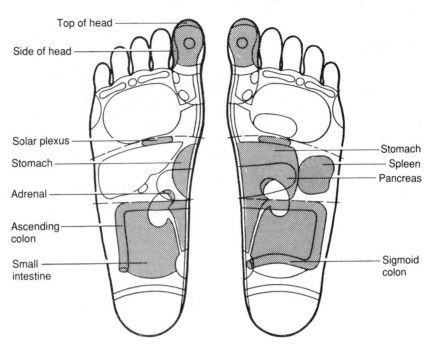

Figure 8.21a *Chart of the soles of the feet showing the reflexes used in treating ME*

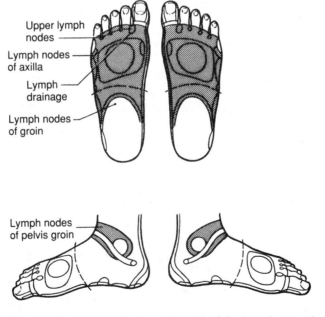

Figure 8.21b *Chart of the tops and sides of the feet showing the reflexes used in treating ME*

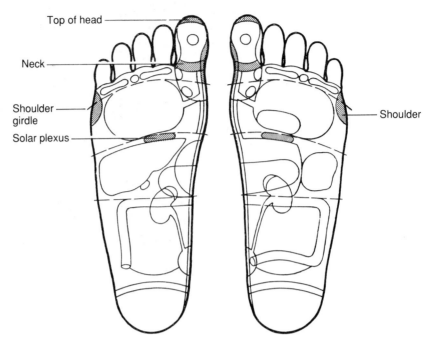

Figure 8.22a *Chart of the soles of the feet showing the reflexes used in treating neck pain*

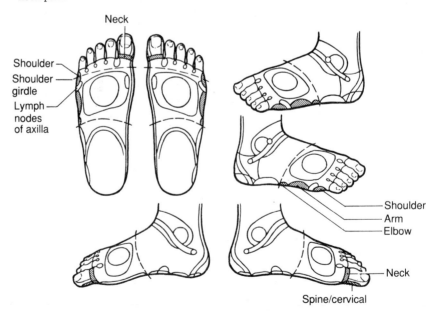

Figure 8.22b *Chart of the tops and sides of the feet showing the reflexes used in treating neck pain*

Pain in the neck region may also be due to a problem with the upper part of the spine and, as a result of neck problems, other problems such as migraine and hearing problems can result.

DR: neck, cervical upper spine (see Figures 8.22a and b).
AR: shoulders, shoulder girdle, arms (as tension can spread to these areas), solar plexus (for relaxation), head (if headaches), ears (if ear problems) - see Figures 8.22a and b.

Psoriasis

Psoriasis is a skin condition the symptom of which is raised red patches covered with silvery scales appearing on the skin. Many parts of the skin may be affected or just an isolated area and normally the affected part will not itch but is usually considered to be unsightly by the sufferer. The causes may be dietary, hormonal or stress related.

DR: area of skin affected (see Figure 8.23).

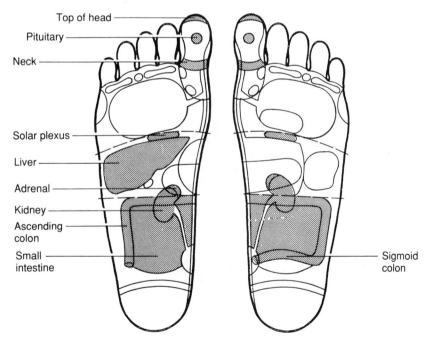

Figure 8.23 *Chart of the soles of the feet showing the reflexes used in treating psoriasis*

AR: adrenals (for inflammation), solar plexus (for relaxation), kidneys (for elimination), small and large intestine (for elimination), liver (for removal of toxins), pituitary (for hormone balance) - see Figure 8.23.

Sciatica

In the condition of sciatica the sciatic nerve becomes inflamed. This nerve - the largest in the body - arises from the lumbar and sacral nerves and extends down across the buttock and down the leg and pain can be experienced along the whole pathway of the nerve or just in certain areas.

The cause of this problem usually stems from the lower spine, but may also involve the pelvis or swelling in the abdomen such as a result of pregnancy or obesity.

DR: sciatic loop and sciatic area up back of ankle (see Figures 8.24a and b).
AR: spine (lumbar and sacral), sacro-iliac joint, pelvic muscles, hips, knees (for parts that can be affected), solar plexus (for relaxation) - see Figures 8.24a and b.

Shingles

The condition of shingles is caused by a virus that affects the peripheral nerves, causing great pain along the nerve and the appearance of small blisters on the surface of the skin supplied by the nerve. The blisters disappear fairly quickly but pain can persist for a considerable time in the part affected. Normally it appears in the upper part of the body, such as across the chest or down the arm, but the face can also be involved.

DR: part affected (e.g., face, chest, arm) - see Figure 8.25b.
AR: lymphatics, spleen (for infection), adrenals (for inflammation), solar plexus (for relaxation) - see Figures 825a and b.

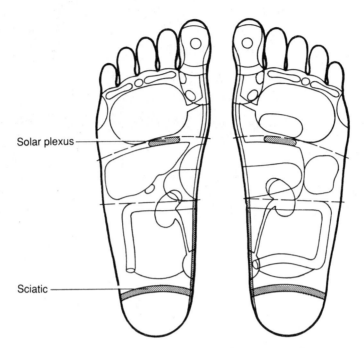

Figure 8.24a *Chart of the soles of the feet showing the reflexes used in treating sciatica*

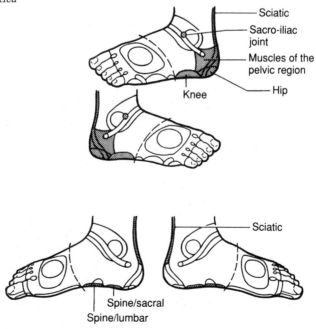

Figure 8.24b *Chart of the sides of the feet showing the reflexes used in treating sciatica*

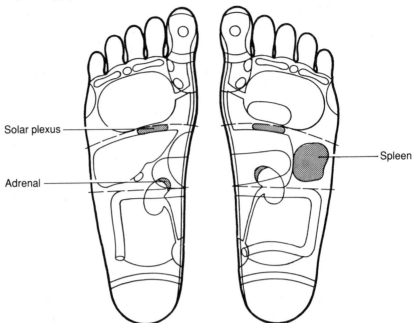

Figure 8.25a *Chart of the soles of the feet showing the reflexes used in treating shingles*

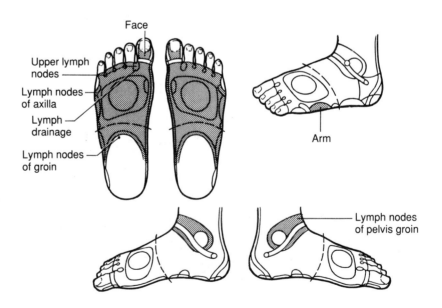

Figure 8.25b *Chart of the tops and sides of the feet showing the reflexes used in treating shingles*

Shoulder Pain

Pain in the shoulder may be due to tension and stiffness in the muscles, a pulled muscle or a condition such as a frozen shoulder where the shoulder becomes stiff and painful so that the arm cannot be moved.

Except where the problem results from a direct injury to the joint or surrounding area, most shoulder problems can be traced to tension in the neck and upper spine. In addition to the shoulder problem, the arm may also be affected.

DR: shoulder and shoulder girdle (see Figure 8.26b).
AR: neck, cervical spine, arm, elbow, solar plexus (for relaxation), adrenals (for inflammation) - see Figures 8.26a and b.

Sinusitis

Sinusitis is inflammation of the sinuses and may occur following a cold or in association with chronic catarrh. There may be pain in the face around where the sinuses are situated, such as the cheekbones and behind the eyebrows, the nose will usually be blocked though sometimes it is runny. The voice can also become husky.

DR: sinuses (see Figure 8.27a).
AR: nose, face, head, eyes, throat, ileo-caecal valve (for excess mucus conditions), small and large intestines (for elimination), adrenals (for inflammation), upper lymphatics (if infection present) - see Figures 8.27a and b.

Stress

Stress and tension are probably the most common causes of many of today's illnesses. The body is able to cope with a certain amount of stress because of the activity of the adrenal glands, but, if these are called on too much, then the body will no longer be able to cope.

The effects of stress are many, but it may give rise to such

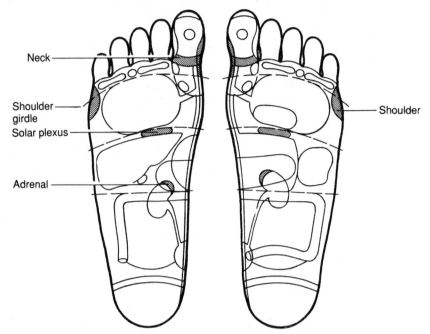

Figure 8.26a *Chart of the soles of the feet showing the reflexes used in treating shoulder pain*

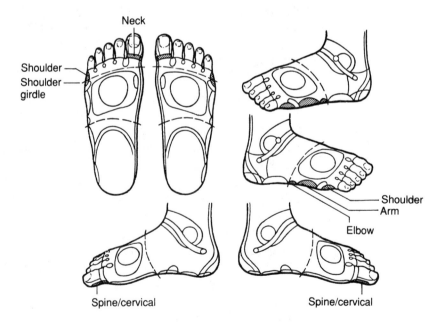

Figure 8.26b *Chart of the tops and sides of the feet showing the reflexes used in treating shoulder pain*

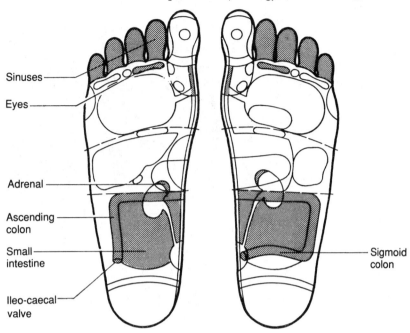

Figure 8.27a *Chart of the soles of the feet showing the reflexes used in treating sinusitis*

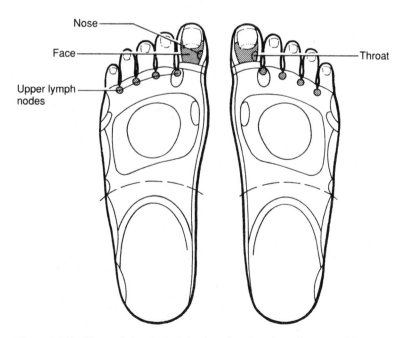

Figure 8.27b *Chart of the tops of the feet showing the reflexes used in treating sinusitis*

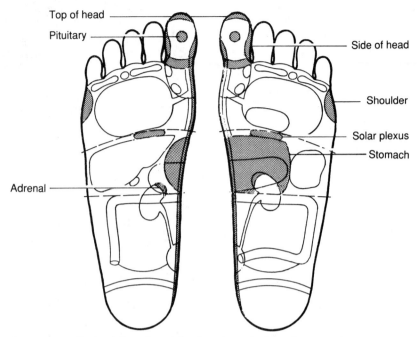

Figure 8.28a *Chart of the soles of the feet showing the reflexes used in treating stress*

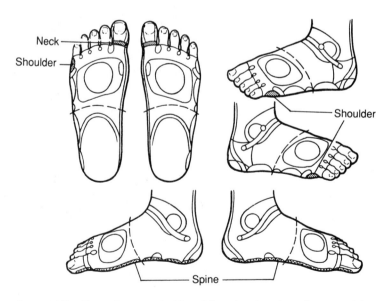

Figure 8.28b *Chart of tops and sides of feet showing the reflexes used in treating stress*

conditions as migraines, digestive upsets, stomach ulcers or skin problems. Stress can also upset the general functioning of many of the parts of the hormonal system of the body.

DR: parts where symptoms present (e.g., head, neck, shoulders, spine, stomach, skin) - see Figure 8.28.
AR: adrenals (for stress), solar plexus (for relaxation), pituitary (for hormonal balance) - see Figures 8.28a and b.

Thyroid Problems

Imbalances in the functioning of the thyroid gland are quite common, with either overactivity or underactivity occurring. There may also be the presence of a goitre (an enlargement of the thyroid gland) and this may be visible in the front of the neck.

With overactivity there is a speeding up of many processes, leading to nervousness, anxiety, sweating, palpitations, weight loss and protruding eyes.

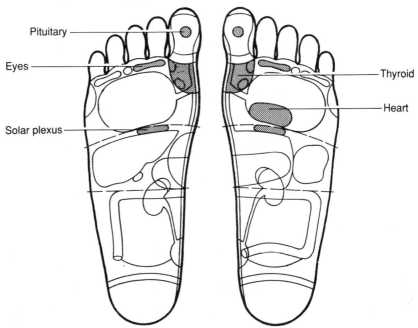

Figure 8.29 *Chart of the soles of the feet showing the reflexes used in treating thyroid problems*

With underactivity there is a slowing down of many processes, leading to sluggishness, tiredness, weight gain and feeling cold.

The approach to treatment using reflexology is the same in cases of overactivity and underactivity as the treatment works to balance the functioning of the gland.

DR: thyroid (see Figure 8.29).
AR: pituitary, heart (for circulation), solar plexus (for relaxation), eyes (if affected by overactivity) - see Figure 8.28.

Tinnitus

For sufferers of tinnitus noises are experienced in the ear that can be variously described as buzzing, hissing or pulsating - the exact sound being different for each person. The cause of the condition can not always be established, but it may be linked to congestion from catarrh, ear infection or damage to the nerve supply to the ear.

This can be a very stressful condition and to many sufferers, the noise experienced becomes louder when all around is quiet, making relaxation and sleep difficult.

DR: ears (see Figure 8.30).
AR: Eustachian tube, side of head, neck, cervical spine, sinuses (if catarrh present), solar plexus (for relaxation), adrenals (for inflammation and stress) - see Figures 8.30a and b.

Varicose Veins

Varicose veins are veins that become enlarged, twisted and swollen. They are usually found in the legs as this is the furthest point from the heart to which the blood has to be returned. The condition is often seen in people who have to stand for long periods or in cases of obesity or during pregnancy where additional weight is being carried. In some cases there may be a disorder involving the valves found in the veins.

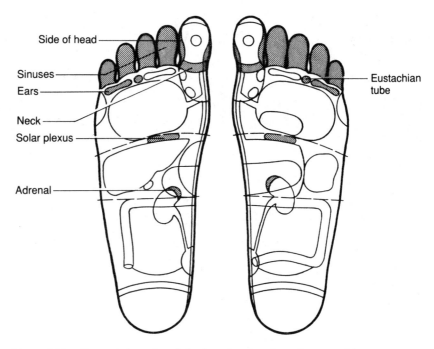

Figure 8.30a *Chart of the soles of the feet showing the reflexes used in treating tinnitus*

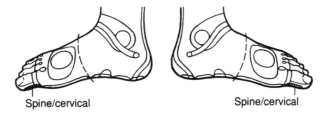

Figure 8.30b *Chart of sides of the feet showing the reflexes used in treating tinnitus*

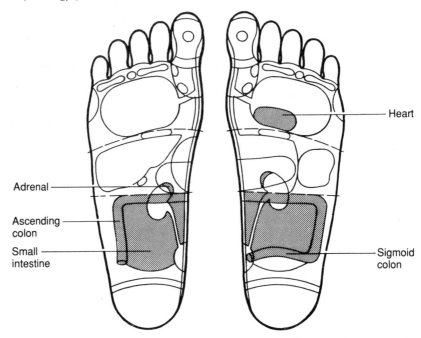

Heart

Adrenal

Ascending
colon

Small
intestine

Sigmoid
colon

Figure 8.31a *Chart of the soles of the feet showing the reflexes used in treating varicose veins*

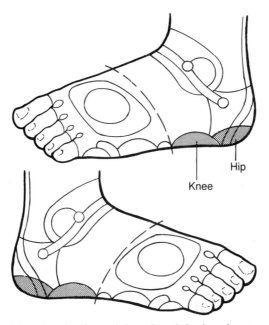

Hip

Knee

Figure 8.31b *Chart of the sides of the feet showing the reflexes used in treating varicose veins*

Although it is unlikely that reflexology treatment will clear varicose veins that are present, it may be effective in helping to prevent further such veins forming and also in easing any pain experienced in the veins.

DR: area affected (e.g., for legs, hips and knees reflexes) - see Figure 8.31b.
AR: heart (for circulation), adrenals (for inflammation), small and large intestine (for elimination) - see Figure 8.31a.

9 *Other Times Reflexology Treatment is Helpful*

In previous chapters, the approach to the treatment of many common conditions, some of which are specific to women and others that affect both men and women, have been looked at. There are, of course, many other conditions that occur, some of which are short term and not serious and some of which are more long-term disorders or more serious. Apart from those instances given on page 46 when reflexology treatment is not appropriate, benefit can be obtained in the treatment of a very wide range of conditions, including some of the more longstanding or serious disorders.

Disorders of The Immune System

There appears to have been a great increase in the number of infections people suffer from and these can lead to a variety of problems in the body. The immune system is there to fight possible infections and prevent them from causing trouble in the body, but if it is not in good working order, then infections can set in and be difficult to clear. It is, therefore, most important to have a strong, healthy immune system.

What the Immune System Does

In response to infection, the body will defend itself locally by the process of inflammation and also throughout the body by building up immunity. Most organisms that get into the body stimulate the white corpuscles in the blood, specifically the lymphocytes, to produce substances called antibodies and antitoxins that react with these toxic organisms and destroy them. The organisms then act as antigens, stimulating antibody formation. The lymphocytes are a type of white blood cell produced in the spleen and the lymph glands. There are two main types: B-lymphocytes, which produce antibodies to counteract bacterial toxins, and T-lymphocytes, which destroy foreign cells by direct contact. The latter are activated in the thymus gland in the body.

The lymphatic system in the body is like a secondary circulatory system with lymph vessels situated throughout the body. This system acts as a drainage and filtering system to prevent bacteria and malignant cells from entering the general circulation. Along the lymphatic vessels are sites known as lymph nodes and the main sites of lymph glands in the body are in the regions of the head and neck, the armpit, the elbow, the groin and the knee. These nodes help to localize infection and so those closest to the site of infection will be most active. For example, with a throat infection, the cervical lymph nodes in the neck will be important and may well become enlarged. Also involved with the lymphatic system are the spleen, the thymus, the tonsils, the adenoids, the appendix and the lymph follicles found in the small intestine.

Infections

For those with infections or a tendency to suffer from infections, working on the lymphatic system reflexes will help strengthen the immune system in the body and therefore help it to overcome the infection present and be more ready to fight future infections. If the immune system is strong, then the body is less likely to succumb to infection.

The lymphatic reflexes are found on the top of the foot with the reflexes for the upper lymph nodes found at the roots of the toes and leading down the top of the foot to the reflexes for the lymph nodes of the groin found over the top of the ankles (see Figure 9.1). The spleen and thymus reflexes are found in the soles of the feet will also be important (see Figure 9.2). The areas are also present similarly in the hands, with the lymphatic reflexes found on the backs of the hands (see Figure 9.3) and the spleen reflex being found in the palm of the left

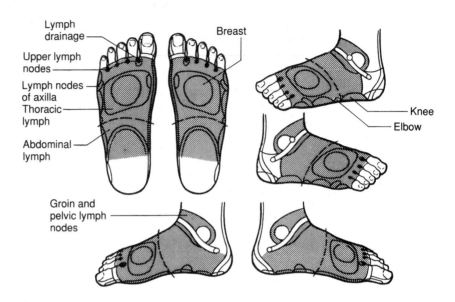

Figure 9.1 *Chart of the tops and sides of the feet showing the reflexes for the lymphatic system*

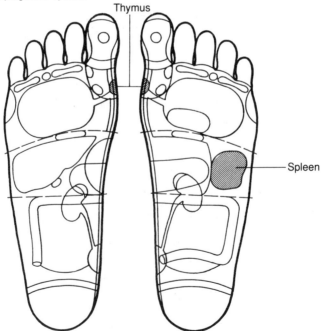

Figure 9.2 *Chart of the soles of the feet showing the spleen and thymus reflexes, important for the lymphatic system*

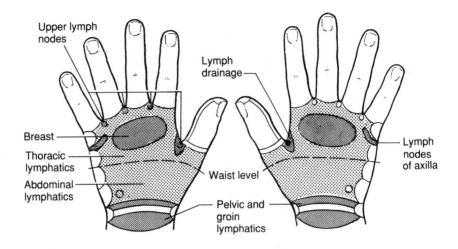

Figure 9.3 *Chart of the backs of the hands showing the reflexes for the lymphatic system*

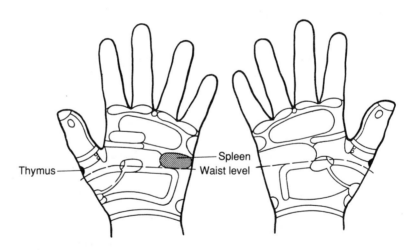

Figure 9.4 *Chart of the palms of the hands showing the spleen and thymus reflexes, important for the lymphatic system*

hand (see Figure 9.4). Work should also be done on the reflexes for the areas of weakness in the body, which are where the infections tend to occur, such as the ear reflex for ear infections, the nose and sinuses reflexes for colds, the bladder reflex for bladder infections.

Cancer

One of the most widespread modern illnesses that causes great concern to people is the condition of cancer. This condition can affect many different parts of the body. A healthy immune system will give the body added strength in fighting the development of cancer cells and so the lymphatic reflexes in the foot and the hand are particularly important.

Reflexology treatment, unlike some other forms of treatment, does not appear to spread cancer cells throughout the body and so therefore can be given to those suffering from cancer to help the body overcome the disorder. If a person is undergoing medical treatment in the form of radiotherapy or chemotherapy for their condition, then there is, unfortunately, always the possibility of unpleasant side-effects occurring and reflexology can be helpful in such instances in reducing the severity of the side-effects. It will also be very relaxing, which is a pleasant contrast to these other treatments.

There are many instances of those who have recovered from cancer who then receive reflexology treatment in order to re-establish a healthy body system to, hopefully, prevent further cancer cells from developing in the future and this is a very wise approach.

Apart from the reflexes for the lymphatic system and the spleen, reflexes that relate to the parts of the body affected and to any specific symptoms that present themselves will be important, together with the solar plexus reflexes for relaxation and the adrenal gland reflexes to help with inflammation and stress.

AIDS

Another condition where the immune system is involved is AIDS - acquired immune deficiency syndrome. Sufferers of this condition have in their bodies the virus HIV, which may lie dormant, not producing significant symptoms, but that may then attack the body, giving rise to the condition of AIDS.

With the great spread of this disorder in recent years and the present lack of successful means for treating the condition, natural therapies can be of some help in trying to keep those who have recently found out that they are HIV positive healthy. For those whose condition has developed, then treatments such as reflexology may be helpful in relieving some of the symptoms and thus maintaining the general well-being of the person.

The important reflexes to treat will be those of the immune system - namely the lymphatic system and the spleen reflexes - together with the reflexes for the solar plexus for relaxation, the liver for detoxification and the adrenals for helping with stress. Other reflexes may also be important depending on the specific symptoms an individual presents.

ME

The condition of ME mentioned in the last chapter, also stems from a weakness in the immune system and so working on the appropriate reflexes (see page 93) can often be beneficial in helping to clear the virus from the system.

Disorders of the Nervous System

What the Nervous System Does

The nervous system controls and integrates the functions of the body, being able to receive and respond to messages from both outside and inside the body and to transmit messages to and from the coordinating centres in the body.

The central nervous system consists of the brain and the spinal cord that, in turn, is linked to the tissues and organs of the body by a peripheral nervous system that is made up of sensory and motor nerve fibres. The sensory nerves carry messages from the tissues and organs to the central nervous system and the motor nerves carry messages from the central nervous system to the tissues and organs. In addition there is also the autonomic nervous system, which consists of sympathetic and parasympathetic systems that help to maintain a stable environment in the body.

The main reflexes that are worked on if there is some dysfunction of the nervous system or simply to maintain it in good working order are shown in Figures 9.5, 9.6, 9.7 and 9.8.

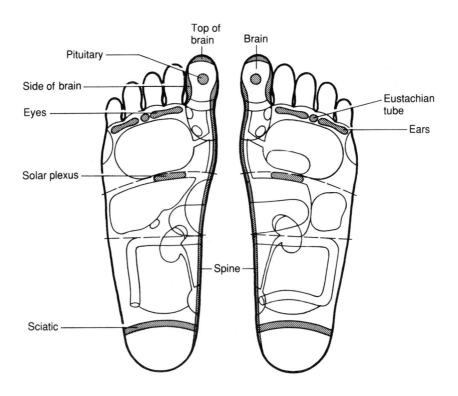

Figure 9.5 *Chart of the soles of the feet showing the reflexes for the nervous system*

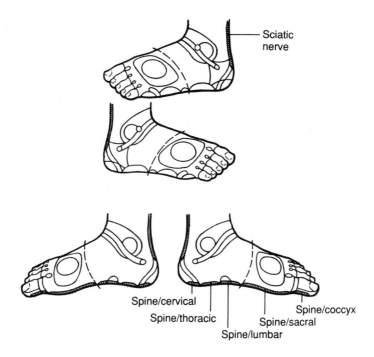

Figure 9.6 *Chart of the sides of the feet showing the reflexes for the nervous system*

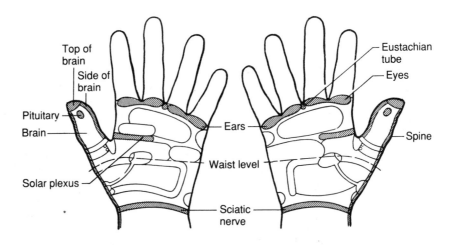

Figure 9.7 *Chart of the palms of the hands showing the reflexes for the nervous system*

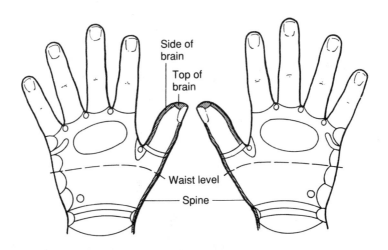

Figure 9.8 *Chart of the backs of the hands showing the reflexes of the nervous system*

Strokes, Parkinson's Disease and Multiple Sclerosis

In conditions such as these where the nervous system is affected, reflexology can be of some help in alleviating the symptoms and, sometimes, in halting the further progress of the condition.

In such conditions, the reflexes for the head and brain and spine will be the most important. As with many conditions where the nervous system is affected, the functioning of the limbs will be impaired and these areas can be treated through the reflexes for the arms (shoulders, arms, elbows) and legs (knees, hips - see Figures 9.9, 9.10, 9.11 and 9.12). In addition there can often be such symptoms as constipation and loss of bladder control, which cause additional distress for the patient, and these symptoms do often respond very well to reflexology treatment. In these instances the reflexes for the intestines (see Figures 9.19, 9.20, 9.21 and 9.22) and the bladder (see Figures 9.13, 9.14, 9.15 and 9.16), respectively, will be important.

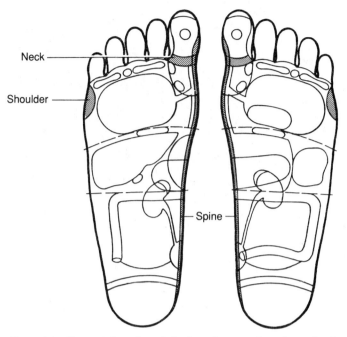

Figure 9.9 *Chart of the soles of the feet showing the reflexes for the musculo-skeletal system*

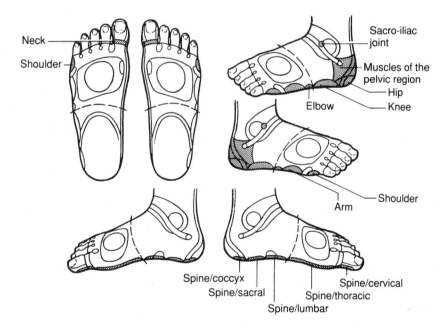

Figure 9.10 *Chart of the tops and sides of the feet showing the reflexes for the musculo-skeletal system*

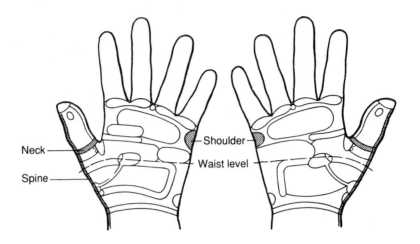

Figure 9.11 *Chart of the palms of the hands showing the reflexes for the musculo-skeletal system*

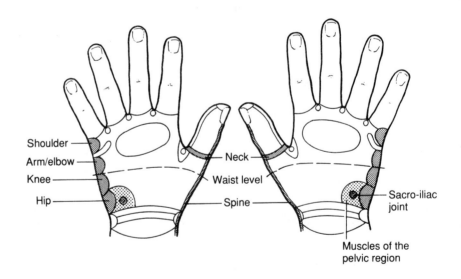

Figure 9.12 *Chart of the backs of the hands showing the reflexes for the musculo-skeletal system*

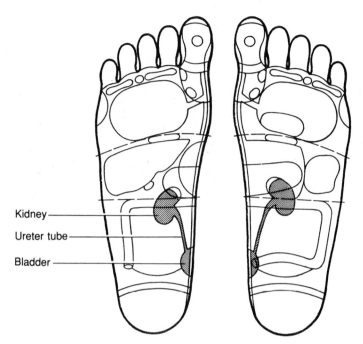

Kidney
Ureter tube
Bladder

Figure 9.13 *Chart of the soles of the feet showing the reflexes for the urinary system*

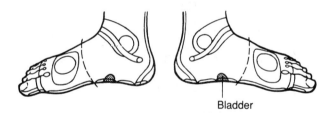

Bladder

Figure 9.14 *Chart of the sides of the feet showing the reflexes for the urinary system*

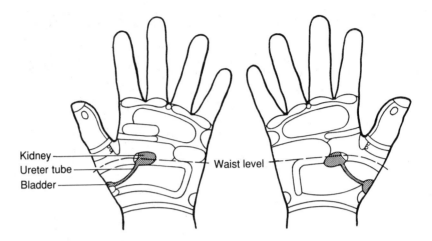

Kidney
Ureter tube
Bladder
Waist level

Figure 9.15 *Chart of the palms of the hands showing the reflexes for the urinary system*

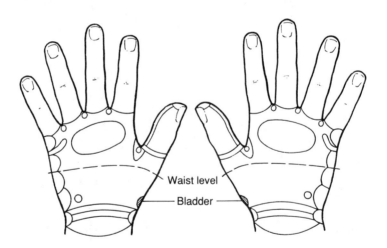

Waist level
Bladder

Figure 9.16 *Chart of the backs of the hands showing the reflexes for the urinary system*

Disorders of the Heart and Circulatory System

What the Heart and Circulatory System Do

Good blood circulation is most important as it is the means by which the various parts of the body receive nutrients and gases such as oxygen and by which waste products are removed. The heart is the pump responsible for ensuring that the circulation is effective. Oxygenated blood leaves the left side of the heart and travels through a system of arteries to the tissues of the body. Here the blood vessels (capillaries) transport such substances as oxygen to the tissues and waste products, including carbon dioxide, away from the tissues. The deoxygenated blood then returns to the right side of the heart via the system of veins. The heart is also connected via the pulmonary circulation to the lungs so that oxygen uptake and carbon dioxide elimination can be achieved.

Good blood circulation is essential to the healthy functioning of all parts of the body and thus, too, is the healthy functioning of the heart.

Heart Conditions

With heart conditions, although treatment has to be given with *extreme care*, improvements to the overall blood circulation throughout the body can be achieved by reflexology treatment and this may help to prevent other problems developing. For example, reflexology can be helpful for problems such as angina and possibly also in cases such as arteriosclerosis (where the arteries are becoming furred up with cholesterol and other deposits).

There are certain instances when it is inappropriate to give reflexology treatment for heart and circulatory problems, however, and these are mentioned on page 46. In all other cases, a good general treatment to all the reflex areas is required, with special attention being given to the heart reflex in the left foot and hand (see Figures 9.17 and 9.18).

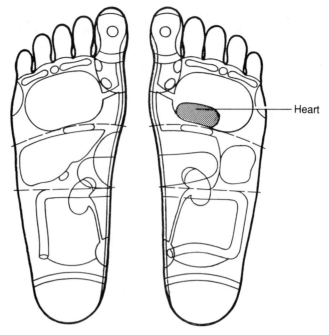

Figure 9.17 *Chart of the soles of the feet showing the reflex for the heart*

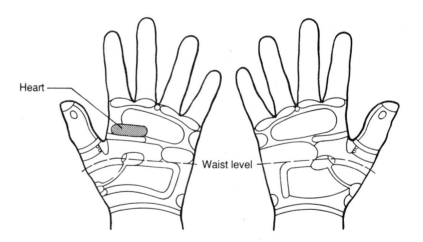

Figure 9.18 *Chart of the palms of the hands showing the reflex for the heart*

Eating Disorders

Losing Weight, Anorexia and Bulimia

There has been much publicity about eating disorders and there is a general trend anyway, particularly among women, to seek ways in which to lose weight. There is no easy way in which to do this, but in many instances controlling the amount and type of food eaten is the best method, which does, however, require a great deal of self-control. Often this is easier if people join a slimming group of like-minded others so that the problems being experienced can be shared and sympathized with and solutions offered.

Reflexology is not a simple, quick way in which to help people lose weight, but, in some cases, it can be found that, together with reformed eating habits, a course of reflexology treatment may have a balancing effect on the body and encourage the various systems to work more efficiently. Apart from the reflexes given in Figures 9.19, 9.20, 9.21 and 9.22, working on the reflexes for the thyroid gland, which controls the metabolic rate of the body can be beneficial as, in some instances, weight gain can be linked to the underactivity of this gland. The pituitary gland reflexes will be important as well as this gland controls the activity of the thyroid gland. Also, by working on the bladder and kidney reflexes, fluid retention may be relieved and massaging the intestinal reflexes will help to ensure that constipation is avoided. In addition, when people are trying to lose weight, the relaxing effect of the treatment will be appreciated and simply the support received from a sympathetic practitioner can help.

The more serious conditions of anorexia nervosa and bulimia do require specialized help, but this can be reinforced and complemented by reflexology treatment to good effect.

Healthy Hair and Nails

Healthy hair and nails are a reflection of good health and, by the same token, if these are in a poor condition, then this is often linked to dietary factors. However, when the general

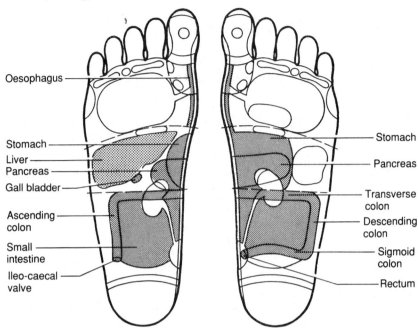

Figure 9.19 *Chart of the soles of the feet showing the reflexes for the digestive system*

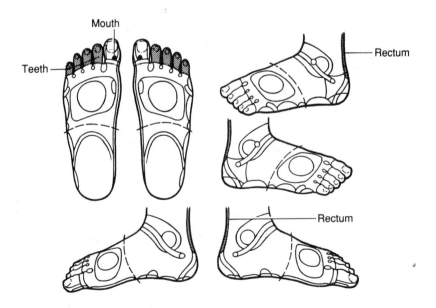

Figure 9.20 *Chart of the tops and sides of the feet showing the reflexes for the digestive system*

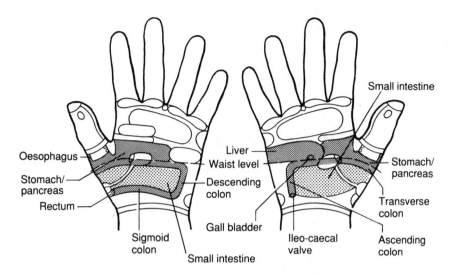

Figure 9.21 *Chart of the palms of the hands showing the reflexes for the digestive system*

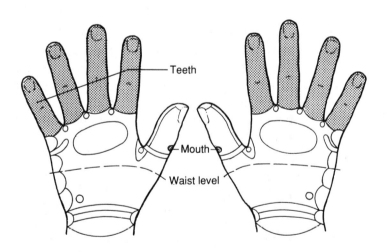

Figure 9.22 *Chart of the backs of the hands showing the reflexes for the digestive system*

health is improved by a course of reflexology treatment, people often see an improvement in the condition of both their hair and nails. One lady reported that since having a course of reflexology treatment her hair had become much thicker and another lady reported that her hair had become curly again!

Giving Up Smoking

Reflexology practitioners are often asked if this form of treatment can be used to help people to give up smoking. As with dieting, reflexology treatment is not a magical answer to this problem, but, certainly where positive steps are being taken to stop smoking, reflexology may be helpful in that it has a relaxing effect and, as a result, people often feel so much better in themselves that, possibly, the *desire* to smoke is reduced (see Figures 9.23, 9.24, 9.25 and 9.26 for the reflexes for the respiratory system).

Coming Off Drugs and Medication

For people trying to come off drugs or wanting to reduce medication, obviously it is important that this takes place under medical supervision. However, as long as *great care* is taken, reflexology treatment can be of use during these times, particularly in terms of its effects of relaxation, increased well-being and improvement in the ability of the body to clear toxins from its various systems.

Foot Problems

Surprisingly often, people think that because reflexology treatment involves working on the feet that the treatment is intended to cure foot problems. This, however, as you will have no doubt realized by now if not before, is not strictly correct; a chiropodist, osteopath or orthopaedic specialist are the best people to see for foot problems. This said, people sometimes find that reflexology treatment does help their foot problems as the general relaxing effect of the massage on the feet helps reduce any tension present in their feet and also loosens up any

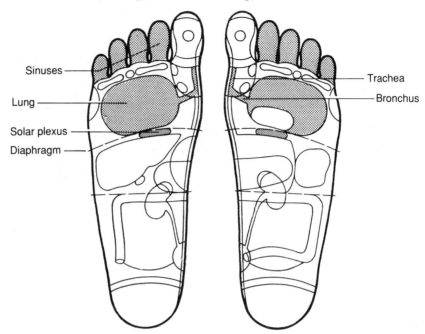

Figure 9.23 *Chart of the soles of the feet showing the reflexes for the respiratory system*

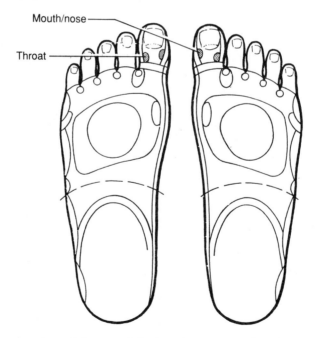

Figure 9.24 *Chart of the tops of the feet showing the reflexes for the respiratory system*

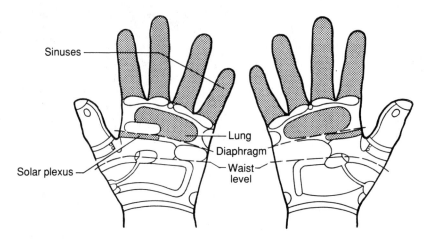

Figure 9.25 *Chart of the palms of the hands showing the reflexes for the respiratory system*

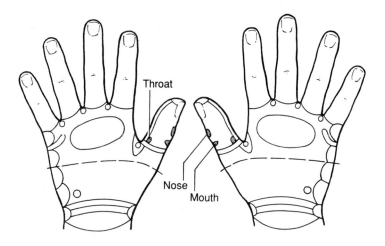

Figure 9.26 *Chart of the backs of the hands showing the reflexes for the respiratory system*

stiff joints there. In addition, different areas of the feet can be treated by massaging the zone-related areas found in the hands if it is not possible to apply treatment directly to the feet for whatever reason.

Am I Too Old or Too Young for Treatment?

Reflexology treatment is suitable for *all* age groups and so can prove beneficial for children through to the elderly. There is no minimum or maximum age limit for treatment.

Treatment of Children

It is usually found that children either strongly like or dislike reflexology treatment, but for those who enjoy the treatment and can sit quietly for the length of time it takes to give the treatment, the benefits will be great. A treatment session to the feet of a child will last for only about 30 minutes as the feet are smaller and so the reflex areas to be massaged are correspondingly smaller. A treatment session to the hands will, therefore, take even less time. A definite pressure can be used on each reflex point, but the pressure used needs to be lighter for a very young child.

When treating children, it is usually not possible to get the feedback required as to which reflexes are tender and which are not - a child will often either say that *all* the points are tender or that *none* are tender. It is therefore important to know which reflex points are the most important for the condition being treated. In general it is found that children respond to treatment very quickly and this is most probably due to the fact that the conditions have not been present for so long and that there are not so many imbalances present in the systems of the body.

The ailments commonly affecting children that can be greatly helped by reflexology treatment include such things as frequent coughs and colds, eczema, asthma and recurring ear infections. The treatment of such conditions is the same as that given in Chapter 8 and the benefits to children of relief from these conditions can be great in that the children will be healthier resulting in less absence from school and a more cheerful disposition.

For the usual illnesses of childhood such as mumps, measles, chicken pox and so on, in the early stages of these conditions it is not really appropriate to give reflexology treatment and the body should be given a chance to overcome the condition itself. However, once improvement has begun, this can be enhanced by a general reflexology treatment, paying special attention to the lymphatic system, spleen and thymus reflexes.

Note that care should be taken when treating children around the age of puberty as often the reflexes are quite tender due to the changes in the hormonal levels in the body and the various physical changes that are taking place.

Treatment of the Elderly

As people get older the likelihood of the systems of the body becoming less efficient increases and therefore illness can occur. If treatment is regularly given to elderly people, therefore, it can be of great benefit to them in helping to keep the various systems of the body working efficiently.

By working on the lymphatic reflexes, the immune system can be strengthened, thus preventing infections setting in. Also the correct functioning of parts such as the bladder and bowels to ensure healthy elimination can be maintained. The general effect of treatment and work on the heart reflex in particular helps the heart to function well and also improves the blood circulation, which tends to become more sluggish with age.

If the condition of diabetes occurs, then this can be helped by working on the pancreas reflex, but particular care must be taken if the patient is on medication for this condition.

Working on the ear reflexes may help to prevent hearing loss and, similarly, working on the eye reflexes may help prevent the eyesight failing. Working on the brain reflexes may help to prevent failing memory. Where there are arthritic conditions, working the appropriate reflexes can be helpful in reducing pain and inflammation, thus aiding mobility.

Stress and Tension

Probably the most common cause of all disorders affecting the body, stress and tension, are experienced by so many people following today's modern hectic lifestyle. It is so important to learn to cope with these everyday stresses in order to prevent illness from occurring. Headaches, migraine, neck pains, backache, asthma, skin problems, hormonal problems and digestive problems are just some of the many that can be caused by stress and tension. Many different forms of relaxation are now known and certainly reflexology treatment has a major role to play as a means of relaxation. There are few people who experience reflexology treatment who do not feel relaxed afterwards, if only for a short while.

An overall treatment is going to help relax all the different parts of the body and particular treatment to the solar plexus and diaphragm reflexes is helpful since these are helpful for relaxation. Also the reflexes to the adrenal glands are important since one of their many functions is to help the body to cope with stress. If the body is subjected to excessive stress, then the adrenal glands become overworked and cannot function as well as they should.

Obviously the relaxation aspect of the treatment can be appreciated to a greater extent when treatment is being given to one by another but self-treatment can also have a relaxing effect. The fact that a treatment to the feet will take nearly an hour is a good thing as it means that there is a longer time to relax. Nowadays people feel so guilty just doing nothing so by having to do nothing for an hour whilst the feet are worked on is often a more acceptable reason for doing nothing and eliminates the guilt feelings which in turn can result in more tension. Putting aside time to relax should certainly not make one feel guilty and in the long term could be a life-saver or extender.

10 *Case Histories*

Amenorrhoea

Miss A was a 16-year-old girl who had had her first period at the age of 11, but, after having 3 periods, these had stopped. Miss A was a very slim young girl who worked very hard at school and was anxious to do well in order to get a place at university. It appeared that stress was probably the primary cause of her problem because, apart from the absence of periods, she was generally in good health, except for an occasional migraine, which occurred about once during each school term.

At the first reflexology session, the feet were fairly sensitive in a number of areas, including the reflexes for the head, neck, lower spine, thyroid, solar plexus, adrenals, ovaries and uterus.

At the second session, Miss A said that following the first treatment she had had quite a bad headache and had felt very tired, but this had passed by the end of the next day. Again, at this session the feet were fairly sensitive, particularly in the same areas as before and a similar response to the treatment occurred.

At the fifth session, Miss A reported that she had had a period that had lasted for four days following the fourth treatment. She seemed very relieved that this had happened and had obviously been worried about not having regular periods like her friends.

Treatments were continued at weekly intervals for ten weeks and a month after her first period, another period occurred. Also, since the first few treatments, she had had no further headaches.

Miss A was very pleased with the reflexology treatment she had received and said that if she had any further problems she would definitely have reflexology again. She thought that it might be sensible to come for treatment before she took her A levels as she did find the sessions very relaxing.

PMS

Miss P was 25 and had always suffered from premenstrual tension in the form of severe abdominal pains for three to four days prior to the start of her period, together with breast discomfort. She also found that during the week prior to the onset of menstruation, she would become depressed and seemed to make a lot of mistakes at work. Her doctor had put her on the contraceptive pill to try to overcome these problems, but this had caused her to put on weight so she had decided to stop taking this form of medication. Her menstrual cycle was regular, with menstruation occurring every 30 days, and for the rest of her cycle she was fit and happy.

When the first reflexology treatment was given, Miss P was about half-way through her menstrual cycle. The reflexes in the feet were quite sensitive, but particularly those to the pituitary gland, thyroid gland, ovaries and uterus. The stomach reflex was also sensitive and Miss P said that she had had stomach ache all day, following a rather spicy meal the evening before.

At the second treatment session, the same reflexes were tender again, except for the stomach, indicating that this had shown up as a direct result of the food she had eaten and that there was not otherwise a problem there.

At the third treatment session, Miss P reported that her premenstrual symptoms were present and that she was experiencing a lot of abdominal and breast pain, though she did not think that she was feeling quite as depressed as she sometimes did at this time. The tender reflex areas were as they had been at the previous sessions, but this time also included the breast, head/brain and solar plexus reflexes.

At the time of the fourth treatment session, Miss P was menstruating so her premenstrual symptoms had passed.

A further ten treatments were given either weekly or fortnightly, depending on when Miss P could fit in an appointment. The premenstrual symptoms were reduced before her second period during this time and prior to her third period, there was only slight abdominal pain and breast discomfort and few signs of depression.

Miss P was delighted with the improvement as the condition had been affecting her life-style, but that if the symptoms continued to be so slight, life would be much easier.

Infertility

Mrs I came for treatment because she seemed to be having difficulty in conceiving. She was 25 years old, had had no history of period problems, was in good health and ate sensibly, but, for the past 2 years she and her husband had been trying to conceive without success. They had both had hospital tests and no problems were found that could account for this failure. Mrs I had been recommended by a friend to try reflexology, so she thought that she would, having heard what a very pleasant treatment it was.

At the first session, her feet were not particularly sensitive, except for the sinus reflexes and after this session Mrs I reported experiencing cold-like symptoms that lasted a few days.

After the second session, Mrs I reported increased elimination from the bowels even though she was not aware that her diet had included anything she did not usually have.

After the third session, Mrs I had several spots on her face, which was most unusual as her skin was usually clear.

After the fourth, fifth and sixth sessions no strong reactions occurred.

Before the seventh session, Mrs I telephoned to say that she had found out she was pregnant and was absolutely delighted.

It appears that the reactions to the initial treatments were healing reactions and that once these unwanted toxins had been cleared from the body, the energy systems were more balanced and conception occurred. An additional reaction to each treatment session was a feeling of being more relaxed, which can only have helped her.

The Menopause

Mrs M was 55 years old and had been through the menopause, with her periods ceasing about 2 years previously. During this time the only problem that had really troubled her had been hot flushes as they would cause her to wake several times in a night, drenched in sweat, and could also embarrass her during the day. In addition, for as long as she could remember, Mrs M had suffered from catarrh and constipation.

At the first reflexology session, Mrs M did not show much sensitivity in the reflex areas in her feet, but particular attention was paid to the reflexes relating to the hormonal system, the sinuses, head and large intestine.

At the second session a week later, Mrs M said that she had noticed no real difference, except that she felt more relaxed and calm in herself. The reflexes were much more responsive at this session with tenderness being felt particularly in the areas relating to the pituitary, sinuses, ileo-caecal valve and sigmoid colon and the reflexes for the ovaries and the uterus.

At the third session, Mrs M said that for a couple of days after the last treatment her nose had been streaming and she thought she might have been getting a cold, but then this stopped and she had felt much clearer in the head. She had also had fewer hot flushes and had a daily bowel movement, which was most unusual for her.

Mrs M completed a course of six treatments, each treatment being given at weekly intervals. After these treatments the hot flushes had stopped, her catarrh had largely cleared and her constipation was no longer a problem. Mrs M decided to come for treatment every four to six weeks in the future to ensure that these problems did not recur.

Fibroids

Miss F was in her late thirties when she came for reflexology treatment for the continual menstrual-type bleeding she was suffering every day, and had been for about six months. During this time it had been necessary for her to have several blood transfusions because of the blood loss. She had been to see a specialist who could find nothing wrong but had suggested that it might be best if she had a hysterectomy. Miss F was not keen to have such a major operation so decided to give reflexology a try.

At the first treatment session, nearly all the reflex areas in both feet were extremely tender and so only a very gentle treatment could be given.

On returning a week later for her second treatment, Miss F delightedly reported that the bleeding had stopped the day after her first treatment. At the second session her feet were far less sensitive and particular attention was given to the reflexes associated with the hormonal system.

At the third session, Miss F reported that she had suffered a very heavy blood loss the day after the last treatment and had been admitted to hospital. She had had to have a blood transfusion, but, after this heavy loss, stopped bleeding again and had been much better since. It had been decided that she must have had fibroids in her uterus but that these had dispersed for some reason.

Miss F continued with treatment for about a year. After the first eight treatments, when she came once a week, the interval between treatments was gradually extended so that, eventually, she came for treatment once a month. After the first month, her periods had returned to normal. She had just a light amount of bleeding at the time of menstruation and she commented that she had forgotten what a normal period was like. This improvement was greatly appreciated and prevented the need for a hysterectomy. Miss F also reported an overall improvement in her health.

Back Pain

Mrs B had experienced recurring bouts of pain in her lower back since she had injured her back while on a boating holiday ten years previously. At the time of the injury she had been given a course of physiotherapy treatment over several weeks and this had eased the pain, but several times a year, she found that the pain returned and it was severe. She had not been able to find a way to stop this. Most of the time she had some pain in her lower back but otherwise, Mrs B was healthy except for a degree of tightness in her neck and shoulders.

At the first reflexology session, great tenderness was found in the reflex areas relating to the neck, shoulders, lower spine (especially on the right side) and the right sacro-iliac joint. Also, the big toe joints appeared very stiff when they were rotated.

After the first session, Mrs B reported that she had felt very tired; she had gone home and slept for two hours and added that it was very unusual for her to sleep in the middle of the day. She had also felt less pain in her back.

The feet were still very tender in the same areas at the second session.

At the third session, Mrs B reported another good week with much less pain in her back and she also felt much freer around the neck and shoulders.

A course of six treatments was given, after which time, the back pain had cleared and the neck and shoulders were still feeling much improved. It was interesting to note that by the end of the course of treatments, the toe rotation exercise had become much easier to do, which corresponded to Mrs B's reports of a loosening up of the neck area. Mrs B was very pleased as she had begun to think that she would have to put up with the persistent pain but now realized she would not have to. She said that if her back troubled her again or if her neck and shoulders became tense again, she would definitely get in touch for further reflexology treatment.

Insomnia

Mrs I had been suffering from insomnia for a year. In the past she had never had a problem sleeping, but, during the past year, she had found herself having difficulty getting off to sleep and was then waking several times in the night. She had tried various things to help her sleep but with no success and most nights only managed about four hours of sleep at the most, which was leaving her feeling very tired during the day. She did not seem to have any major problems she was worrying about that would explain her disturbed sleep pattern. Her work as a secretary to a company director in a small business was demanding and she had quite a high degree of responsibility, but she did not feel that she was worrying about her job.

The first treatment session took place one evening and Mrs I came straight from work. Her feet were rather stiff and there were several areas of hard skin and a bunion on the right foot, which she said had probably resulted from wearing fashionable shoes that were a bit too tight for her feet. There were not many tender reflex points in the feet, but slight tenderness was felt when those to the neck, head, upper and lower spine were worked on. By the time the left foot was being worked on, Mrs I kept dropping off to sleep and by the end of the treatment session she felt very tired. It was recommended that if she still felt very tired when she got home that she should go to bed immediately and try to sleep.

At her next visit, Mrs I said that she had gone to bed when she got home and had slept for six hours. During the week she had found that she was not waking so much in the night, but was still having great difficulty in going off to sleep.

Treatments were given at weekly intervals and, by the fourth treatment, Mrs I was able to report a few nights of good sleep. After six treatments, Mrs I was quite delighted that the problem of insomnia was now hardly evident and she was managing to go to sleep most nights as soon as she got to bed and was not waking in the night – sleeping straight through for about seven hours. Her family had commented that she seemed more interested in them again now that she was sleeping better.

Allergic Rhinitis and Asthma

Miss R was a 30-year-old woman who, for many years, had suffered from allergic rhinitis. She seemed to be allergic to many things and her symptoms made it look like she had a perpetual cold. Hospital tests had confirmed the evidence of an allergic reaction to many common substances and so she tried to avoid these substances as much as possible, but it was not easy. The condition was particularly bad during the hay fever season as pollen was one of the worst of her allergies.

Apart from the rhinitis, Miss R was reasonably healthy, though she did tend to suffer from digestive problems fairly frequently and also occasional attacks of asthma for which she was on medication.

Miss R's feet at the first session felt rather moist and warm, even though it was not a warm day. Nearly all of the areas of the feet showed some tenderness, but particularly the regions relating to the sinuses, eyes, large intestine, kidneys and adrenals. The area relating to the lungs felt rather tight. During the treatment, Miss R blew her nose constantly and her eyes streamed, but, apparently, this was not any worse than normal.

At the second treatment session, Miss R said that she had felt very relaxed after her previous treatment, but that her symptoms had remained the same. Again, the reflexes were sensitive throughout the treatment of both feet.

At the third session, Miss R appeared to blow her nose less and did say that this had been the case during the previous week.

At the fourth session, Miss R reported a great improvement, saying that she had blown her nose much less and that her eyes had not been watering.

After seven treatment sessions, given at weekly intervals, the condition had cleared almost completely.

Treatments were continued every four to six weeks and the condition remained greatly improved. Miss R continued with the sessions to ensure that her problem did not return and also because she found the sessions so relaxing. Even during the hay fever season, when she would normally have been at her worst, the symptoms did not reappear. Another improvement was with regard to her asthma. Since starting reflexology treatment, she had not had an asthma attack and very rarely felt the need to use her medication. In addition, she found that she was suffering fewer digestive upsets.

Eczema

Miss E was a 6-year-old who had developed eczema over most of her body at about the age of one. Her parents had tried her on a diet eliminating cow's milk and, although this had helped considerably, there were still patches of eczema in the creases of the elbows, the wrists and behind the knees and also sometimes on the face. The skin itched a lot, causing Miss E to scratch and aggravate the condition and she was very self-conscious about the state of her skin, particularly in the summer months when the affected parts were not covered by clothes.

Miss E was a bit fidgety when treatment first started and was perhaps rather nervous about what was going to be done to her. However, she settled down during the session. As is often the case when treating children, Miss E did not report that any particular reflex points were tender, but a good general treatment was given.

A course of four treatments at weekly intervals was given and by the second treatment there was already a slight improvement in the condition of the skin. This improvement developed further with each treatment. By the fourth treatment, the skin was almost clear and Miss E said how much she enjoyed her foot treatments.

Several months later, Miss E's mother rang to say that her daughter's eczema was now completely clear and had not deteriorated at all since she had finished the course of reflexology treatment. She was most grateful to have been introduced to reflexology and said that if any of her family developed any problems in the future they would certainly give reflexology a try.

Thyroid Problems and Constipation

Mrs T booked a course of treatment sessions for a number of problems. Her husband had recently died after a year of serious illness and she was now feeling very run down, depressed and tired. For the last three years she had been suffering from an overactive thyroid gland, for which she was now taking a low dose of medication. She also suffered from chronic constipation, sometimes not having a bowel movement more than once a week. This problem she thought was probably linked to her diet, which contained very little roughage. She also admitted to being rather a fussy eater, not eating very much at any meal, including few fruits or vegetables in her diet and having a preference for white bread rather than brown. She had tried recently to improve her diet but had really not enjoyed doing so.

At the first treatment session, her feet were rather tense and showed many tender reflexes. The most tender reflexes were those for the pituitary gland, thyroid gland, head and brain areas (Mrs T also said that she suffered occasionally from migraines, which she thought were stress related), neck and shoulder areas (due to tension), solar plexus and both the small and large intestine areas, in particular the reflex for the sigmoid colon. Mrs T felt very relaxed by the end of the treatment and had nearly fallen asleep.

At subsequent treatments, the same reflex areas continued to appear to be tender, but Mrs T began to see an improvement in herself. She felt less tense and was also having a bowel movement at least every other day.

A course of six treatments at weekly intervals was given and then Mrs T decided to come for treatment once a month because she was so pleased with the improvements and wanted to maintain this. In addition, when she next had a blood test to check her thyroid, the results showed that there was no further need for medication and Mrs T felt certain that this improvement was due to her regular reflexology treatment.

11 Caring for Your Feet and Hands and Other Therapies Involving Foot and Hand Treatments

Knowing about the presence of the reflex areas in the feet and hands, which represent the whole body brings about the realization of just how important the feet and hands are. The feet have the important task of supporting the body and making it possible to walk, run and jump and the hands perform the vital tasks of touching, holding and carrying. As we have seen, though, as well as helping us with these daily tasks, they are also a reflection of the body and how healthy, or otherwise, it is. It is possible, therefore, that any damage to the foot or hand may affect the reflex area there, which, in turn, might cause a problem in the part of the body to which it corresponds. Thus, care of the feet and hands is essential to the health of the rest of the body.

Caring for Your Feet

Normally people pay much more attention to their hands than to their feet as the hands are on view for most of the time. They will be washed more frequently and creams will be massaged into them to soften the skin far more frequently than creams will be massaged into the feet, even though the feet have to do a great deal of work also.

It is most important to care for the feet, too. Regular washing followed by thorough drying - in particular between the toes - is an essential part of good foot care. After washing, the gentle massage of a moisturizing cream into the feet will keep the skin of the feet smooth. The toe nails should also be kept cut short and that of the big toe in particular should be cared for so that an ingrowing toe nail does not develop. In some instances this can be the cause of headaches as the ingrowing nail will be pressing on the head reflex.

It is important that sensible shoes are worn most of the time to ensure no damage to the foot and in this respect men tend to be kinder to their feet than women as most men's shoes follow the natural shape of the foot. The occasional wearing of high-heeled shoes may not do much damage, but regularly wearing them can result in more serious problems. Not only will the high-heeled shoes affect the overall posture of the wearer, but they can also affect the Achilles tendon up the back of the leg. In this region are found the reflexes for the sciatic nerve, rectum and uterus, all of which may possibly become affected.

Hard Skin and Callouses

Where hard skin and callouses have developed, these should be regularly attended to with a pumice stone or similar to remove the layers of dead skin and then extra moisturizing cream applied. Note that, contrary to popular belief, it is much easier to remove hard skin when the feet are *dry* than when they are wet.

If there is a large amount of hard skin, then the professional help of a chiropodist should be sought to remove this. After it has been removed, though, there will be a tendency for hard skin to develop in the area again if it is not looked after properly. The best way to keep the hard skin at bay is to regularly soak the feet in warm water to which a small amount of, for example, an oil has been added. This can be followed by further moisturizing of the skin of the feet.

Although it feels good, regularly using talcum powder on the feet after washing is not a good idea as this tends to clog the pores in the feet and will also tend to dry out the skin of the feet. Foot baths, however, which massage the feet in addition to soaking them in water, can be quite relaxing and beneficial to the circulation in the feet.

Where there is a build-up of hard skin on the foot, as well as treating it, the possible cause should be looked for to avoid it recurring. It may well have resulted from pressure on the foot due to ill-fitting or fashionable shoes or poor posture, whereby the weight of the body has not been distributed evenly on the foot.

Interestingly, it is sometimes found that there is a build-up of hard skin over a reflex area on the foot that directly relates to a part of the body that is not working correctly. For example, there may be a build-up of hard skin over the ball of the foot, which is where the lung reflex is to be found and the person may then have a lung problem, such as asthma.

Bunions

One of the most common foot problems is bunions. A bunion is an inflamed joint and the joint most affected is that where the first metatarsal joins the phalange of the big toe on the inner side of the foot. The most likely cause of this is the wearing of shoes that are too tight and, because more women wear constricting fashionable shoes than men, more women suffer from bunions than men. However, bunions can also be found in conjunction with a problem with the thoracic region of the spine or the thyroid gland as the reflexes for these areas are found in this part of the foot.

Athlete's Foot and Verrucas

For the same reasons given above, it is important for common conditions such as athlete's foot and verrucas to be noticed and treated. There are many natural products now available for the treatment of such conditions, including the use of tea tree oil, which has recently grown in popularity for such problems and can be quite effective.

Again, it is possible that where such a problem exists on the foot, there may be a problem in the area of the body that corresponds to the affected reflex area of the foot. An example of this effect comes to mind. A lady started suffering from migraines at the same time that a crop of verrucas developed over the tip of her big toe. Once the verrucas had been cleared from the area, and this took quite some time, the migraines ceased.

Other Therapies Involving Foot and Hand Treatments

There are forms of treatment other than reflexology that involve working on the feet and the hands, but the methods used are different; the precise form of massage used in reflexology treatment is unique to reflexology. Some of these treatments are purely aimed at correcting foot or hand problems, but others, like reflexology, are treatments aimed at having an effect on the whole body via areas of the feet and hands.

Acupressure

Acupressure follows a similar system of meridian lines to acupuncture, but pressure using the fingers rather than needles is applied at the pressure points. As with acupuncture, because the meridian lines extend to the feet and hands, treatment of these areas may be involved together with treatment of other parts of the body.

Acupuncture

Acupuncture is a form of ancient Chinese medicine based on a system of energy lines in the body through which flows the life force, *ch'i* in Chinese. There are 14 major channels of energy running through the body and these are called meridian lines. Each is named according to the organ or function connected to its energy flow and the meridian lines are divided into positive and negative forces - Yang and Yin respectively. The Yang lines begin at the top of the head, face and fingertips and descend towards the centre of the body and towards the earth. The Yin lines start from the toes and the centre of the body and ascend to the head and the fingertips. Of the 12 Yang and Yin meridians, the 6 Yang meridians flow along the lateral aspect of the arms and legs, face and back and the 6 Yin meridians follow along the inner aspect of the arms and legs and the pelvic and thoracic regions. In the foot, the Yin meridians are

those of the kidney, liver and spleen and the Yang meridians
are those of the bladder, gall bladder and stomach. In the hand,
the Yin meridians are those of the lung, heart and heart
constrictor and the Yang meridians are those of the small
intestine, large intestine and triple heater. The two vessel line,
the Yang Governing Vessel Meridian and the Yin Conception
Vessel Meridian control the energy flow along all the meridian
lines and govern their activities.

To treat using acupuncture, needles are applied at various
pressure points along the meridian lines in order to balance the
flow of energy. As pressure points are given on the feet and
hands, treatment may involve needles being inserted at these
points as well as into other parts of the body.

Aromatherapy

In aromatherapy, treatment involves the use of essential oils
that are derived from natural plant sources. Different plant
essences are known to be helpful for different disorders and an
appropriate blend of oils will be massaged into the body during
an aromatherapy treatment.

An initial diagnosis is given to determine which oils will be
required and this can be carried out by an analysis of the spine,
but often a short reflexology massage is given as the means of
diagnosis. By finding which parts of the foot are tender it can
be ascertained which parts of the body are out of balance and
then the appropriate essential oils can be selected to treat these
imbalances.

Chiropody

Chiropody is the treatment of foot disorders and although the
term podiatry, strictly, means foot surgery, it is usually
interpreted as being just the American word for chiropody.

A chiropodist will deal with common problems, such as
ingrowing toe nails, corns, callouses, verrucas, and will also be
able to advise on the ways in which the build-up of callouses
can be avoided and help with the correction of conditions
affecting the actual structure of the foot. In general, the

chiropodist does not perform surgery on the foot, although there are an increasing number of chiropodists qualified to do so. More usually, surgery would be performed by an orthopaedic surgeon.

Herbalism

Herbalism is another form of natural treatment that has been used for thousands of years. Treatment involves taking herbs either in the form of medicines or teas, when they are to be taken internally, or extracts, which are rubbed into the skin, used as compresses, added to baths or used as poultices.

There are some herbalists who will use the herbs required for a specific condition in foot baths, the healing benefits of the herbs being absorbed through the feet. This method became popular due to the work of the French herbalist Maurice Messegue, working in the early part of the 1900s.

Massage

A complete body massage will include massaging the feet and hands. Massage can be a very relaxing form of treatment, as noted with regard to reflexology, as well as helping to reduce the tension that can build up in various muscles.

The hands are used to give the massage and a variety of techniques are used, different ones being appropriate to the different regions being treated. Although the work done on the hands and feet during a full body massage will be more general than it would be during a reflexology session, the principle of helping the whole body through the hands and feet will still apply.

The Metamorphic Technique

The metamorphic technique was developed by Robert St John who had studied reflexology with the late Doreen Bayly and then developed the method along different lines.

The reflex area for the spine found along the inner side of each foot he linked to the gestation period - the nine months from conception to birth. He felt that during the pre-natal period, the physical, mental, emotional and spiritual characteristics became established and that energy blocks occurring during this time could affect the development of the person. With the metamorphic technique, therefore, massage is given using a lighter pressure than is used for reflexology treatment, the tips of the fingers working over the area in a circular, light rubbing movement. Work commences on the big toe areas and particularly the upper and lower corners of the nail relating to the pineal and pituitary glands and then down the spine reflex and up the back of the heel. Massage is also given under the inner ankle bone across the top of the foot to below the outer ankle bone, which is where the reflex for the pelvic girdle is located. About 30 minutes is spent working on each foot in these areas. The right foot is worked first as it relates to patterns that a person is establishing in the present and determines what a person is making of their life, while the left foot relates to patterns not yet expressed but which have been present since the person came into being. In addition, massage may be given to the head and also to the hands with the hands being worked in a similar manner to the feet.

This method sometimes brings about good results when used in the treatment of mentally retarded children, but it can also be helpful in a wide range of other disorders affecting all ages.

Polarity Therapy

Polarity therapy was first described by Dr Randolph Stone in the 1940s and involves a method of treating the body to stimulate and balance its life energy. It was developed from the method of zone therapy described by Dr Fitzgerald (see page 153) and involves balancing the electromagnetic energy currents that flow backwards and forwards between the positive and negative poles of the body.

The head is considered to be positively charged and the feet negatively charged, so energy tends to flow from the head to the feet. Because the feet are changeover points, where the flow of energy is reversed, the feet are considered to be of great importance.

In addition to the ten longitudinal zones described by Dr Fitzgerald, Dr Stone also described the existence of nine horizontal zones in the body, with six of these being found in the feet and hands. Each of these zones has a positive, negative and neutral charge and there is a link between these areas in the same horizontal zone.

The method of polarity therapy does not involve precise massage of reflex points, but the hands are placed on the body to redirect the energy flow. Some practitioners incorporate the principles of polarity therapy into their reflexology treatment sessions.

Shiatsu

Shiatsu is very similar to acupressure and could be considered to be the Japanese version of this. The word 'shiatsu' is Japanese for 'finger pressure' and with this method pressure is applied at pressure points, or *tsubos*, found along the meridian lines. Some of these pressure points are located on the feet and hands so treatment may be given to these areas.

Vacuflex Reflexology

The vacuflex system of reflexology was developed by a Danish practitioner, Mrs Inge Dougans. The feet are placed in large felt boots that cover the whole foot and the ankle. Air is then removed from the boots using a vacuum pump, which creates equal pressure all over the feet and, at the same time, massages all the reflex points in both feet with an equal pressure. After about five minutes, the boots are removed and markings and discoloration will be seen on the feet over the reflex areas that are out of balance.

After diagnosing any problems using the boots, treatment is given using suction pads placed over acupuncture meridian lines along the lower legs and arms to help balance the energy flow in the body and release blockages. This second part of the treatment lasts for about 20 minutes. This method has similarities to reflexology treatment, but is a little more mechanical in its approach.

Zone Therapy

Zone therapy was, you will recall, described in Chapters 2 and 3 as it is the method from which reflexology evolved and, in many instances, the term is used for the same method used in reflexology. However, whereas reflexology treatment will involve working on the reflex points found in the feet or hands, zone therapy will involve working on points found throughout the body along the ten longitudinal zones described by Dr Fitzgerald as well as the other areas of the body that he further subdivided, such as the head and the ear, for which there are a further ten zones. Also, in zone therapy a much firmer pressure is used to work on the various pressure points and often gadgets are used to exert the pressure.

A Note On These Therapies in Relation to Reflexology

Several of the methods mentioned above show similarities to reflexology treatment and are working towards balancing energy flow in the body. Whether one is working on the same energy system though has yet to be established.

As with reflexology, many of these methods, with the exception of chiropody, which is very specific, can be helpful in the treatment of a wide range of disorders that can affect the whole body and therapists practising in each of these therapies can give examples of the benefits that can be achieved in many different cases. It would be wrong to say that any one therapy is more effective than another as each will have its own value. In some cases it may be that when one form of treatment is used, aspects of similar treatments will also be involved, sometimes unknowingly. The most important factor is that practitioners of each of the therapies mentioned are trying to restore and maintain good health for the patient following an holistic approach.

12 *Summary*

From the preceding pages it will be clear to you just how very wide the range of benefits reflexology treatment can offer is. It has already been mentioned that the method cannot always help everyone, but, for most conditions, there is a good chance that the treatment will help to some extent at least. If you are interested in trying reflexology treatment, then it is worth doing so by visiting a practitioner, as it is unlikely to do any harm and it may well do a lot of good.

In many instances, following a course of treatment, conditions may clear up completely and this improvement should be permanent unless outside factors cause a recurrence of the condition. Where improvement is partial, then there is often an alleviation of symptoms and this can prove to be a bonus in itself, especially when there is relief from pain, feelings of relaxation and greater well-being. Indeed, these last two benefits are sometimes vital for self-healing to occur in the body, so they can lead on to later improvements in the condition.

Certainly the general effects of reflexology treatment sessions are very valuable. They ensure that there is good circulation in the body, which aids the transportation of nutrients to the various parts of the body and the removal of waste products from the system. Also there are usually improvements in the various eliminatory systems, such as the skin, lungs, kidneys and intestines, and this is beneficial in helping to clear unwanted toxins from the body. The stimulatory and strengthening effect of treatments on the lymphatic system is another benefit as this helps to ward off harmful organisms, preventing infections and the occurrence of disorders involving the immune system.

There are many possible causes of diseases in the body. Some diseases may be hereditary, so that a genetic disorder is inherited from a parent. Some diseases may be *partly* hereditary in that a tendency towards suffering a particular disease is inherited, but that the disease will only present itself if certain environmental factors exist. Some diseases are due to infection, caused when microbes such as bacteria and viruses successfully invade the body. Some diseases are due to deficiency, whether this be of foods, vitamins or hormones. Whatever the cause, however, there is less chance of the body succumbing to illness if it is in a strong and balanced state and this is particularly so when the immune system is strong. The preventive aspect of reflexology treatment is, therefore, very important. This can be reinforced by maintaining a healthy life-style, that is, eating a varied, healthy diet, taking regular exercise, adequate rest and exposing yourself to a minimum of stress.

Reflexology is a safe form of treatment and, if and when necessary, it can be combined with orthodox medical treatment. It can also be combined with other forms of complementary therapy such as homoeopathy, herbalism, osteopathy, naturopathy and aromatherapy. It is probably not appropriate to combine reflexology with treatments such as acupuncture and acupressure as the methods are working along very similar lines. This said, it is important not to have too many treatments at the same time for several reasons.

First, many complementary forms of treatment can cause certain healing reactions to occur. These need time to settle down and for the toxins to be cleared from the system. If too many treatments are given together, then there is the possibility of causing very strong healing reactions that could make a person feel very unwell.

Second, it becomes difficult to assess which treatments are doing good and which are not. It is generally found that a person will find a complementary therapy that they respond well to and if they respond well on one occasion, then there is a likelihood that they will respond well to the same form of treatment on another occasion. Thus, if one form of complementary medicine does not work for a person it need not mean that other forms will also be unsuccessful.

Making the initial decision about which form of treatment to try is usually governed by such things as the availability of practitioners in your area and whether you have had any personal recommendations made to you regarding a particular practitioner or therapy - this latter factor seeming to be the greatest influencer of all.

Sometimes it is found that a person is responding well to a course of reflexology treatment, but that the condition does not disappear altogether and it may well be that, at this stage, giving the person an additional form of treatment is the best option. Some reflexology practitioners, therefore, may use other therapies such as dietary therapy, vitamin therapy, tissue salts or the Bach flower remedies and it may be that the inclusion of one of these just tips the balance towards further improvement. Equally, the reverse situation occurs. It may be that a person trying a course of a treatment such as homoeopathy or herbalism is making good improvement, but needs something a little bit extra to make a full recovery and in these instances reflexology treatment might make the difference. A second therapy would not be considered, though, until the first treatment had been given a fair opportunity to succeed. With all of the natural therapies the approach of treating the person as a whole is always followed, but it may be found that one particular type of treatment is more helpful than another at helping a person at a particular stage of recovery.

Throughout this book the treatment of disorders has been described, but, as mentioned above, reflexology can be used to equally good effect as a means of preventative medicine. You do not need to wait to be ill before having reflexology treatment and, indeed, it is more sensible to have regular treatment as a preventative measure rather than waiting for something to go wrong. In the old days in China, the doctor was only paid when his patients were well. Once they became ill he was seen to have failed in his duty to them. Modern medicine has established the complete reverse of this approach. Natural treatments such as reflexology, however, help to keep the body in balance and working efficiently, so, provided no strong external factors such as poor diet and stress persist, which will be fighting against balance in the body, good health should prevail.

For there to be complete harmony in the body, there needs to be harmony on the physical, mental, emotional and spiritual levels. Although working predominantly on the physical level, reflexology can contribute positively towards achieving harmony in the body on all of these levels and, consequently, the achievement of good health.

Where to Find a Reflexology Practitioner

It is important once you have decided to try reflexology treatment that you see a properly qualified practitioner. There are a number of groups that can provide details of qualified reflexology practitioners and the following addresses should be of use to this end.

Administration Office
The British Reflexology Association
Monks Orchard
Whitbourne
Worcester WR6 5RB
Tel: 01886 21207

The British Reflexology Association, founded in 1985, holds a register of members (price £1.50) that gives the names and addresses of reflexology practitioners throughout Great Britain. The Association can also provide details of reflexology training courses and books, charts and videos as The Bayly School of Reflexology is the official teaching body of the British Reflexology Association (it operates from the same address). Courses are held at London and regional venues and there are branches of the School in Switzerland, Spain and Kenya.

The Institute for Complementary Medicine
P.O. Box 194
London SE16 1QZ
Tel: 0171-237 5165

The ICM operates the British Register of Complementary Practitioners and this has a reflexology section.

The British Complementary Medicine Association
St Charles Hospital
Exmoor Street
London W10 6DZ
Tel: 0181-964 1205

The BCMA has organization councils for the different categories of complementary medicine, including a Reflexology Organisations Council. This consists of representatives from the different reflexology organizations. A list of representative groups is available from the BCMA.

International Council for Reflexology
4311 Stockton Boulevard
Sacramento
CA 95820
USA

Formed in 1981, the Council aims to link reflexology associations and their members world-wide and therefore has contracts with reflexology associations throughout the world. An annual conference is held in the autumn.

Index

HOMOEOPATHY FOR WOMEN

Rima Handley

Homoeopathy is a fascinating and increasingly popular subject, and women in particular are discovering how it can help with very many common problems associated with menstruation, pregnancy and menopause.

Homoeopathy for Women is written by one of the UK's leading homoeopaths, and co-founder of the Northern College of Homeopathic Medicine. It explains:

- the holistic nature of homoeopathy
- how it works
- why it is particularly suited to women's ailments
- what happens when you visit a homoeopath
- how you can use it to improve your own and your family's health
- how to prescribe effectively for simple conditions and first aid

'This accessible and interesting introduction to homoeopathy makes fascinating reading as Rima Handley describes how homoeopathy can benefit women at all stages in their lives: from infancy through to old age'

Miranda Castro F.S.Hom, author of
The Complete Homoeopathy Handbook and
Homoeopathy for Mother and Baby.

HERBAL THERAPY FOR WOMEN

Elisabeth Brooke

More and more women are discovering that herbal remedies can provide natural and effective treatments for their health problems, particularly when orthodox methods fail to help.

Herbal Therapy for Women provides a concise, intelligent introduction to herbs and herbalism. It explains how to prepare teas and tinctures from fresh or dried herbs, which herbs are suitable for healing each ailment, and how herbs can enhance each stage of a woman's life, from puberty to menopause.

Elisabeth Brooke is a qualified medical herbalist who combines teaching with clinical practice.

'Elisabeth Brooke is a herbalist with a strong personal vision, and her approach lends a holistic dimension to the basic herbal format.'
Christopher Hedley, *Member of the National Institute of Medical Herbalists*

'It is exciting to see a woman's herbal written from the perspective of a practitioner with many years experience working "in the field" and one who dares to offer a personal way of practising which inevitably will challenge the status quo.'
Helen Stapleton, *Independent Midwife and Medical Herbalist*

FLOWER REMEDIES
FOR WOMEN

Christine Wildwood

Flower remedies are suitable for people of either sex, as well as animals and plants, but here Christine Wildwood looks at this system of healing from the female perspective. In a celebration of womanhood, she explains how these gentle essences can help a woman through all her rites of passage: the onset of menstruation, pregnancy, childbirth, the menopause and facing up to death.

Flower therapy is not an alternative to other forms of treatment, rather a complementary approach which addresses the emotional, mental and spiritual aspects of our being. *Flower Remedies for Women* relates the development of flower therapy and explains how the essences work and how to apply them. The remedies of Dr Edward Bach are covered in detail and the Californian essences and Australian Bush essences are introduced. Other supportive measures are also included. With these gentle remedies, we may work towards bringing about our own healing and fulfilment.

Christine Wildwood is an aromatherapist who uses flower remedies to aid healing. She is the author of several other books.

HOMOEOPATHY FOR WOMEN	0 7225 2781 0	£4.99 ☐
HERBAL THERAPY FOR WOMEN	0 7225 2722 5	£4.99 ☐
FLOWER REMEDIES FOR WOMEN	0 7225 2842 6	£4.99 ☐
AROMATHERAPY FOR WOMEN	0 7225 2260 6	£4.99 ☐
ACUPRESSURE FOR HEALTH	0 7225 2702 0	£8.99 ☐
SELF MASSAGE	0 7225 2510 9	£7.99 ☐
HEALTHY BY NATURE	0 7225 2803 5	£9.99 ☐
THE JAPANESE WAY OF BEAUTY	0 7225 2976 7	£8.99 ☐

All these books are available from your local bookseller or can be ordered direct from the publishers.

To order direct just tick the titles you want and fill in the form below:

Name: _____

Address: _____

_____

_____ Postcode: _____

Send to: Thorsons Mail Order, Dept 3, HarperCollins*Publishers*, Westerhill Road, Bishopbriggs, Glasgow G64 2QT.
Please enclose a cheque or postal order or your authority to debit your Visa/Access account —

Credit card no: _____

Expiry date: _____

Signature: _____

— to the value of the cover price plus:
UK & BFPO: Add £1.00 for the first book and 25p for each additional book ordered.

Overseas orders including Eire: Please add £2.95 service charge. Books will be sent by surface mail but quotes for airmail despatches will be given on request.

24 HOUR TELEPHONE ORDERING SERVICE FOR ACCESS/VISA CARDHOLDERS — TEL: **041 772 2281**.